# Enhancing Early Child Development

T0235941

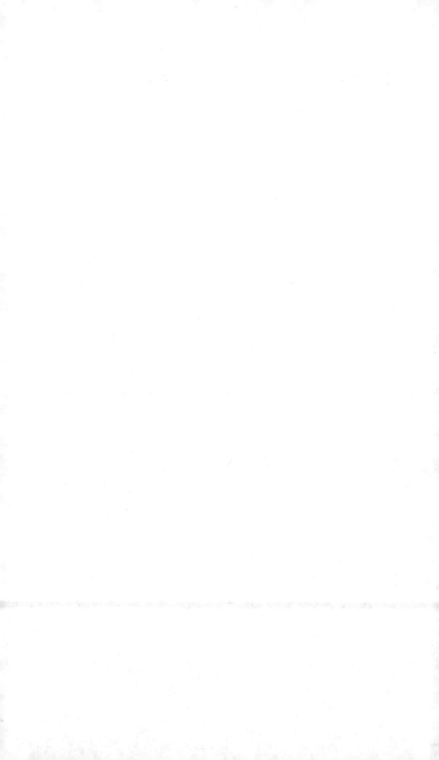

Durriyah Sinno · Lama Charafeddine
Mohamad Mikati

# Enhancing Early Child Development

## A Handbook for Clinicians

With Contributions by:
Rebecca L. Holt, MD
Aravindhan Veerapandiyan, MBBS

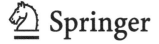 Springer

Durriyah Sinno, MD
Department of Pediatrics and
  Adolescent Medicine
American University of Beirut
  Medical Center
Beirut, Lebanon

Lama Charafeddine, MD, FAAP
Department of Pediatrics and
  Adolescent Medicine
American University of Beirut
  Medical Center
Beirut, Lebanon

Mohamad Mikati, MD
Division of Pediatric Neurology
Duke University Medical Center
Durham, NC, USA

ISBN 978-1-4614-4826-6        ISBN 978-1-4614-4827-3 (eBook)
DOI 10.1007/978-1-4614-4827-3
Springer New York Heidelberg Dordrecht London

Library of Congress Control Number: 2012954288

Printed on acid-free paper

Springer is part of Springer Science+Business Media (www.springer.com)

# Rationale for Developmental Interventions in Children

## Introduction

Early childhood is a critical developmental period during which children undergo physical, cognitive, and emotional growth. Early childhood developmental interventions (ECDIs) have been developed with the aim of improving the overall functioning of children as well as their cognitive and motor skills. ECDIs are based on the fact that young children respond best to specific modalities designed to encourage and stimulate their developmental progress. Such ECDIs include, but are not limited to, educating parents, teachers, and caregivers to enhance their knowledge and practices and delivering services to children that can be home-based, center-based, or a combination of both. This applies to children with neurological conditions as well as to otherwise healthy children. There is currently convincing evidence from both developing and developed countries that ECDIs can make significant differences in the physical, intellectual, social, and emotional development of children [1]. However, implementation and outreach of these programs require making such interventions available to children. At one level, parents and caretakers can deliver many of the interventions if primary care providers can educate them about methods that can improve their child's condition and/or enhance his/her development. This book is intended to be a resource for primary care providers such as pediatricians and even specialists to help them in educating parents and caretakers of children in need of ECDIs. At another level, global implementation of ECDIs requires a collaborative effort of basic scientists, developmental psychologists, primary care providers, parents, policymakers, and local and global communities. In this chapter, we review the rationale for implementation of ECDIs at the local as well as at the global levels. Such rationale is based on ethical considerations, evidence from clinical studies, cost-effectiveness of ECDIs, as well as on evidence from basic science studies.

## Ethical and Legal Rationale

The convention on the Rights of the Child (CRC) provides a global vision of the basic rights of the children, in particular, "the right to survival and development, and to education that develops children's personality, talents, and mental and physical abilities to the fullest" [2]. It stipulates that all children regardless of background should be offered a continuum of care, health care, and education through a multisectorial approach to enable them to exercise their full potential. Every child has the right to develop his or her potential to the maximum extent possible, to become physically healthy, mentally alert, socially competent, emotionally sound, and ready to learn. Early childhood development rights have been increasingly incorporated into international agreements and agendas. According to CRC, one of the most effective ways to ensure that every child reaches his or her full potential is through high-quality ECDIs [2]. The World Fit for Children agenda, United Nations' 10-year agenda that includes 21 goals for children with commitments to child rights, prioritizes early childhood development [3], asserting that nations must promote the physical, psychological, spiritual, social, emotional, cognitive and cultural development of children. The Education for All (EFA) commitments include expansion and improvement of early childhood care and education among goals to be met by 2015 (United Nations General Assembly 2002; United Nations Educational, Scientific and Cultural Organization [UNESCO] 2000) [3]. In addition, the CRC also affirms the rights of children for successful transition to primary school and alternative care.

# Beneficial Effects of Early Childhood Developmental Interventions in Clinical Studies

ECDIs result in short-term improvements as well as long-lasting effects on cognitive skills and other developmental domains not only in impaired children but also in normally developing children.

## *Interventions in Normally Developing Children*

Several randomized controlled studies on ECDI programs in USA have demonstrated that these programs improve cognitive outcomes of normally developing children (Table 1). Early head start programs that were studied including a total of 17 programs (7 home based programs, 4 center based programs and 6 mixed) targeted low income families with children up to 3 years of age and produced significant positive impacts on cognitive development with an estimated effect of 1.6 points higher on the Bayley and 2.1 points higher on the Peabody test in the Head Start group compared to the control group [4]. A program for expectant African-American mothers comprising cognitive stimulation and well-baby care by a pediatrician and home visits by a nurse from birth to 3 years of age resulted in a mean IQ score at age 3 of 8.1 points ($p < 0.001$) higher in children of mothers who were in the intervention group compared to that of the control group [5]. Similarly, an Intellectual stimulation program (Milwaukee project) [6] offered to children living in otherwise deprived environments resulted in higher mean IQ at ages 6, 10, and 14 years in the experimental group compared with the control group [6]. Furthermore, Wasik et al. demonstrated that disadvantaged children at birth because of educational or social circumstances had greater developmental and intelligence scores at 12, 18, 24, 36, 48, and 54 months of age when their parents received either a combined center-based care and family education compared to those children whose parents received family education only [7]. Finally, Olds et al. showed a superior mental developmental scores at 2 years of children whose mothers were enrolled in a periodic home visiting program during pregnancy and from birth to second birthday of the child compared to their counterparts who received routine care [8].

**Table 1** Studies demonstrating beneficial effects in normally developing children

| Country | Intervention | Targeted population (age at enrollment) | Effects |
|---|---|---|---|
| *Early Childhood Developmental Intervention Programs in Unites States of America* | | | |
| USA [5] | Cognitive stimulation program | African–American children (birth) | Increase in IQ |
| USA [6] | Milwaukee project—intellectual stimulation program | Children from deprived environments (birth) | Increase in IQ |
| USA [7] | Center-based and family education | Children at risk for cognitive difficulties (birth) | Increase in cognitive scores |
| USA [8] | Home visiting by nurses and paraprofessionals | Children of women with no previous live births (birth) | Increase in mental developmental scores |
| USA [4] | Early Head Start program (center-based, home-based, or mixed) | Children from low-income families (up to 3 years) | Improved cognitive development |
| *Early Childhood Developmental Intervention Programs in Middle and Low Income countries* | | | |
| Africa [9] | Preschool Programs in Cape Verde and Guinea | Normal children (2–6 years) | Improved cognitive development |
| Africa [12,13] | Madrasa Preschool program | Normal children (3–6 years) | Improved cognitive development |
| Bangladesh [11] | Preschool program | Normal children (4.5–6.5 years) | Increase in cognitive scores |
| Bolivia [10] | Preschool program (PIDI-proyecto Integral de Desarrollo Infantil) | Children from poor families (6 months–6 years) | Increase in cognitive scores |
| India [14] | Anganwadi preschool program | Normal children (4–6 years) | Increase in IQ |
| Mexico [16] | Conditional Cash Transfer Program | Normal children (2–6 years) | Improved cognitive, language, and motor development |
| Philippines [15] | Integrated services of family day care, community-based parent education, and school readiness | Normal children (0–4 years) | Improved cognitive, social, motor, and language development |

A number of studies have shown that preschool programs in developing countries have positive impacts on the cognitive outcome of children: (1) in Guinea and Cape Verde preschool attendance increased the children's cognitive development at 5 years of age by 4.41 points and 7.27 points, respectively [9]. (2) The Bolivian preschool program PIDI (Proyecto Integral de Desarrollo Infantil) in which home-based integrated services were provided to children (6 months to 6 years) of poor urban families resulted in significant positive effect on cognitive and psychosocial test scores of children enrolled in the program compared to those who were not [10]. (3) A cross-sectional study conducted to evaluate the effectiveness of preschool programs in Bangladesh compared the performance of preschool children to those of a control group from villages where there were no preschools. This study revealed better performance on the WPPSI-III of children attending preschool with a modest effect size for vocabulary, verbal, and nonverbal reasoning and large effect size (1.00) for school readiness [11].( 4) The effectiveness of Madrasa preschool programs in Kenya, Zanzibar, and Uganda providing an active learning experience through a culturally appropriate curriculum to children from low socioeconomic backgrounds was compared to other types of locally available preschools in East Africa. The children enrolled in the Madrasa programs were followed up to 4.3, 6, and 7.1 years and were found to have increased cognitive scores by 0.4 standard deviations per year compared to the control group [12, 13]. (5) In India, Ade et al. evaluated the impact of an ECDI package delivered through the Anganwadi preschool centers. This case control study showed significantly higher IQ and DQ values for children in the intervention preschools compared to controls [14]. (6) In addition, in Philippines, Armecin et al. evaluated the effectiveness of an integrated ECDI program consisting of four components: (a) family day care for 3–5-year-old children, (b) community-based parent education, (c) an 8-week school readiness program for children entering formal education, and (d) growth monitoring and improved service of health and nutrition. Their study showed that these integrated services resulted in a substantial improvement at 2 years follow-up in cognitive, social, motor, and language development of children enrolled in program areas relative to nonprogram areas [15]. (7) Finally, a Conditional Cash Transfer program in Mexico (*Oportunidades*), the largest of its kind where a monthly fixed stipend was given to families obtaining preventive care and educational scholarships to children attending school for a minimum of 85 % of the time, showed improved cognitive, language, motor development of children aged 24–68 months [16].

## Interventions in Special Populations

A substantial number of studies addressed the Developmental intervention programs for preterm infants. Spittle et al. [17] performed a Cochrane Review of 16 studies investigating the effectiveness of ECDI programs initiated at birth and continued during the first year of life on cognitive and motor development. This meta-analysis revealed that intervention improved cognitive outcomes of infants at 0–2 years and at the preschool age (3–<5 years); however, the effect was not sustained at school age (5–17 years). A more recent randomized controlled trial in Norway of a modified version of the Mother–Infant Transaction Program for low-birth weight preterm infants showed a significant increase in the IQ scores at 5 years of 7.2 points higher in the intervention group compared to the control group [18]. A USA study providing Toddler–Parent Psychotherapy for depressed mothers showed a decline in IQ at age 3 of children in the nonintervention group while the intervention and control groups maintained their IQ scores [19].

In the West Indies, severely malnourished children were recruited to receive weekly home visits for 3 years or regular care. At 14 years follow-up, children in the intervention group had a significantly higher verbal IQ (by 10 points) and full scale IQ (by 8.6 points) as compared to the nonintervention group [20]. Several early intensive and behavioral interventions such as University of California at Los Angeles–Lovaas-based interventions using applied behavior analysis (ABA), "Early Intensive Behavioral Interventions" (EIBI), and intensive parent training approaches have shown that there are benefits in areas of cognitive, language, social, and adaptive functioning in children with autism spectrum disorders (ASD) [21–23]. Early interventions for children with cerebral palsy have been shown to improve their overall functionality [24–28]. In addition, several studies have demonstrated that aerobic exercises, neurodevelopmental treatment, and constraint-induced movement therapies could impact physiological outcomes and motor development of children with cerebral palsy [29–31]. Early interventions focusing on improving motor skills and language development have been shown to be effective in children with Down syndrome [30, 32, 33]. Likewise children with Duchenne Muscular Dystrophy had positive effect on muscle strength and function and decreased risk of secondary complications including scoliosis, contractures, and impairments of respiratory function after early interventions [26, 34–36].

In brief, the available studies do demonstrate that ECDI programs result in benefits not only in children with medical conditions but also in normal developing children. Despite the limitations imposed by the heterogeneity of these programs, their variable duration and variable length of follow-up, these programs still result in the enhancement of cognitive as well as noncognitive development.

# Cost-Effectiveness of Early Childhood Developmental Interventions

Several studies support the argument that ECDI programs are cost-effective with long-term benefits not only to individuals but also to society as a whole. These studies include, among others, the Perry preschool program, the Title I Chicago Child–parent Centers program and the Carolina Abecedarian project. These studies have demonstrated that, for every dollar spent, there is a benefit to cost ratio of direct and indirect benefits of 7.16, 6.87, and 2.69 fold at the ages of 27, 21, and 22 years, respectively [37]. Similarly, a cost-effectiveness study of a Bolivian preschool program demonstrated a benefit–cost ratio of direct benefits ranging from 1.89 to 2.93 projected to the age of 60 years [10]. These studies have emphasized the gains and savings to society resulting from ECDIs due to reduced crime, reduced grade repetition/grade retention, reduction in welfare payments, improved educational attainments and reduction in children's enrollment into special schools, reduced divorce rates, increase in individual income, higher rates of credit cards holding, and finally increase in tax payments. These studies, however, relied on models that were applied for specific programs in specific situations. We recently have developed an analysis model that can be applied worldwide to estimate the cost-effectiveness of ECDIs using IQ gains resulting from such programs as proxy for subsequent benefits from ECDIs. Our analysis resulted in a cost–benefit ratio of direct benefits of 4.19 at the age of 65 years for interventions done at the age 3 years for 2 years and with a breakeven point at the age of 24 years [38].

## Basic Science Rationale for Early Interventions

Recent advances in developmental neurobiology have demonstrated that brain development can be enhanced by several interventions. Optimal stimulation of the developing brain during critical times creates the foundation for enhanced lifelong skills [39]. The basic mechanism lies in the concept of cerebral plasticity which is the brain's ability to learn, remember, forget, reorganize, and recover from injury [40]. In this section, we summarize our findings from the recently reviewed literature.

An expanding body of basic animal studies demonstrates that cerebral plasticity, therefore development, is enhanced by several interventions including level of parental interaction, environmental enrichment, and nutritional supplements in addition to potential therapeutic modalities as hypothermia, erythropoietin, antidepressants, transcranial magnetic stimulation, transcranial direct current stimulation, and stem cells therapy. Discussion of all modalities is beyond the scope of this book; however, we choose to focus on the parental and environmental factors. Animal studies have shown that environmental enrichment stimulates the two activity-dependent mechanisms underlying cerebral plasticity, neurogenesis, and synaptogenesis in various regions of the brain [41–48]. Environmental enrichment improved learning, memory, auditory function, and exploratory behavior; it restored visual acuity and ocular dominance and reduced reactivity to stress, motor deficits, and seizures [41–48]. Parental level of interaction was studied in rat pups exposed to maternal licking and grooming: The frequency of maternal licking and grooming was shown to enhance learning under basal conditions, alter synaptic structure and function, and result in a differential responsiveness to glucocorticoids and stress [49]. These changes were correlated with a higher expression of brain-derived growth factor (BDNF) [50]. Prenatal choline supplementation has been shown to be protective against the long-term cognitive and neuropathological effects of status epilepticus in adult rats [51–53]. Lastly, foods rich in polyphenols such as pomegranate juice, blueberries, and green tea extract have been shown to protect the neonatal mouse brain against hypoxic-ischemic injury when given to mothers in their drinking water [54]. In addition, long-term omega-3 fatty acid supplementation in rats with epilepsy has been demonstrated to enhance hippocampal neurogenesis and BDNF levels [55].

Durham, NC, USA                    Aravindhan Veerapandiyan
Palo Alto, CA, USA                        Rebecca L. Holt
                                          Mohamad A. Mikati

# References

1. Engle PL, Fernald LC, Alderman H, et al. Strategies for reducing inequalities and improving developmental outcomes for young children in low-income and middle-income countries. Lancet. 2011;378(9799):1339–53.
2. Evaluation of UNICEF'S early childhood development programme with focus on government of Netehrlands funding (2008–2010). Global Synthesis Report. 2011.
3. United Nations General Assembly Convention on the Rights of the Child. Nov 20, 1989. United Nations Treaty Series, Vol. 1577. [http://www.unicef.org/crc/]. Accessed April 2012.
4. Love JM, Kisker EE, Ross C, et al. The effectiveness of early head start for 3-year-old children and their parents: lessons for policy and programs. Dev Psychol. 2005;41(6):885–901.
5. Gutelius MF, Kirsch AD, MacDonald S, Brooks MR, McErlean T, Newcomb C. Promising results from a cognitive stimulation program in infancy. A preliminary report. Clin Pediatr. (Phila). 1972;11(10):585–93.
6. Garber HL. The Milwaukee project: preventing mental retardation in children at risk. Washington, DC: American Association on Mental Retardation; 1988.
7. Wasik BH, Ramey CT, Bryant DM, Sparling JJ. A longitudinal study of two early intervention strategies: project CARE. Child Dev. 1990;61:1682–96.
8. Olds DL, Robinson J, O'Brien R, et al. Home visiting by paraprofessionals and by nurses: a randomized, controlled trial. Pediatrics. 2002;110(3):486–96.
9. Jaramillo A, Tietjen K. Early childhood development in Africa: can we do more for less? Washington, DC: World Bank; 2001.
10. Behrman JR, Cheng Y, Todd PE. Evaluating preschool programs when length of exposure to the program varies: a nonparametric approach. Rev Econ Stat. 2004;86(1):108–132.
11. Aboud FE. Evaluation of an early childhood preschool program in rural Bangladesh. Early Child Res Q. 2006;21(1):46–60.
12. Malmberg LE, Mwaura P, Sylva K. Effects of a preschool intervention on cognitive development among East-Africsn preschool children: A flexibly time-coded growth model. Early Child Res Q. 2011;26(1):124–33.

13. Mwaura PAM, Mohamed BT. Madrasa early childhood development program: making a difference. In: Garcia M, Pence AR, Evans J, editors. Africa's future, Africa's challenge early childhood care and development in Sub-Saharan Africa. Washington, DC: World Bank; 2008:389–406.

14. Ade A, Gupta SS, Maliye C, Deshmukh PR, Garg BS. Effect of improvement of pre-school education through Anganwadi center on intelligence and development quotient of children. Indian J Pediatr. 2010;77(5):541–46.

15. Armecin G, Behrman JR, Duazo P, et al. Early childhood development through an integrated program: evidence from the Philippines. Washington, DC: World Bank; 2006.

16. Fernald LC, Gertler PJ, Neufeld LM. Role of cash in conditional cash transfer programmes for child health, growth, and development: an analysis of Mexico's oportunidades. Lancet. 2008;371(9615):828–37.

17. Spittle A, Orton J, Doyle L, Boyd R. Early developmental intervention programs post hospital discharge to prevent motor and cognitive impairments in preterm infants. The Cochrane Library, The Cochrane Collaboration. 2009(1):1–49.

18. Nordhov SM, Ronning JA, Dahl LB, Ulvund SE, Tunby J, Kaaresen PI. Early intervention improves cognitive outcomes for preterm infants: randomized controlled trial. Pediatrics. 2010;126(5):e1088–94.

19. Cicchetti D, Rogosch FA, Toth SL. The efficacy of toddler-parent psychotherapy for fostering cognitive development in offspring of depressed mothers. J Abnorm Child Psychol. 2000;28(2):135–48.

20. Grantham-McGregor S, Powell C, Walker S, Chang S, Fletcher P. The long-term follow-up of severely malnourished children who participated in an intervention program. Child Dev. 1994;65(2 spec no.):428–39.

21. Dawson G, Rogers S, Munson J, et al. Randomized, controlled trial of an intervention for toddlers with autism: the early start denver model. Pediatrics. 2010;125(1):e17–23.

22. Lovaas OI. Behavioral treatment and normal educational and intellectual functioning in young autistic children. J Consult Clin Psychol. 1987;55(1):3–9.

23. Warren Z, McPheeters ML, Sathe N, Foss-Feig JH, Glasser A, Veenstra-Vanderweele J. A systematic review of early intensive intervention for autism spectrum disorders. Pediatrics. 2011;127(5):e1303–11.

24. Rosenbaum P. Cerebral palsy: what parents and doctors want to know. BMJ. 2003;326(7396):970–74.

25. Russman BS, Ashwal S. Evaluation of the child with cerebral palsy. Semin Pediatr Neurol. 2004;11(1):47–57.

26. Dennis CW, Schlough KA. Gross motor development. In: Hooper SR, Unmansky W, editors. Young children with special needs. NJ: Pearson Education; 2004:224–67.

27. Anttila H, Autti-Ramo I, Suoranta J, Makela M, Malmivaara A. Effectiveness of physical therapy interventions for children with cerebral palsy: a systematic review. BMC Pediatr. 2008;8:14.

28. Pennington L, Goldbart J, Marshall J. Speech and language therapy to improve the communication skills of children with cerebral palsy. Cochrane Database Syst Rev. 2004(2):CD003466.

29. Hoare BJ, Wasiak J, Imms C, Carey L. Constraint-induced movement therapy in the treatment of the upper limb in children with hemiplegic cerebral palsy. Cochrane Database Syst Rev. 2007(2):CD004149.
30. Mahoney G, Robinson C, Fewell RR. The effects of early motor intervention on children with Down syndrome or cerebral palsy: a field-based study. J Dev Behav Pediatr. 2001;22(3):153–62.
31. Rogers A, Furler BL, Brinks S, Darrah J. A systematic review of the effectiveness of aerobic exercise interventions for children with cerebral palsy: an AACPDM evidence report. Dev Med Child Neurol. 2008;50(11):808–14.
32. McLean WE, Hartley SL. Down syndrome. In: Salkind NJ, editor. Encyclopedia of human development Vol I. Thousand Oaks, CA: Sage; 2006:394–96.
33. Valentin-Gudiol M, Mattern-Baxter K, Girabent-Farres M, Bagur-Calafat C, Hadders-Algra M, Angulo-Barroso RM. Treadmill interventions with partial body weight support in children under six years of age at risk of neuromotor delay. Cochrane Database Syst Rev. 2011;12:CD009242.
34. Merlini L, Cicognani A, Malaspina E, et al. Early prednisone treatment in Duchenne muscular dystrophy. Muscle Nerve. 2003;27(2):222–27.
35. Manzur AY, Kuntzer T, Pike M, Swan A. Glucocorticoid corticosteroids for Duchenne muscular dystrophy. Cochrane Database Syst Rev. 2008(1):CD003725.
36. Rose KJ, Burns J, Wheeler DM, North KN. Interventions for increasing ankle range of motion in patients with neuromuscular disease. Cochrane Database Syst Rev. 2010(2):CD006973.
37. Reynolds AJ, Temple JA. Cost-effective early childhood development programs from preschool to third grade. Annu Rev Clin Psychol. 2008;4:109–39.
38. Veerapandiyan A, Alderman H, Steele SU, MA M. Cost-benefit analysis of early childhood development intervention programs. Abstract presented in 40th Annual Meeting of Child Neurology Society. Dec 26–29, 2011.
39. Holt RL, Mikati MA. Care for child development: basic science rationale and effects of interventions. Pediatr Neurol. 2011;44(4):239–53.
40. Hebb D. The organization of behavior. New York: Wiley; 1949.
41. Cao L, Jiao X, Zuzga DS, et al. VEGF links hippocampal activity with neurogenesis, learning and memory. Nat Genet. 2004;36(8):827–35.
42. Johnston MV. Plasticity in the developing brain: implications for rehabilitation. Dev Disabil Res Rev. 2009;15(2):94–101.
43. Kempermann G, Kuhn HG, Gage FH. More hippocampal neurons in adult mice living in an enriched environment. Nature. 1997;386(6624):493–95.
44. Nithianantharajah J, Hannan AJ. Enriched environments, experience-dependent plasticity and disorders of the nervous system. Nat Rev Neurosci. 2006;7(9):697–709.
45. Okuda H, Tatsumi K, Makinodan M, Yamauchi T, Kishimoto T, Wanaka A. Environmental enrichment stimulates progenitor cell proliferation in the amygdala. J Neurosci Res. 2009;87(16):3546–53.
46. van Praag H, Kempermann G, Gage FH. Neural consequences of environmental enrichment. Nat Rev Neurosci. 2000;1(3):191–8.

47. Veena J, Srikumar BN, Raju TR, Shankaranarayana Rao BS. Exposure to enriched environment restores the survival and differentiation of new born cells in the hippocampus and ameliorates depressive symptoms in chronically stressed rats. Neurosci Lett. 2009;455(3):178–82.
48. Yang J, Hou C, Ma N, et al. Enriched environment treatment restores impaired hippocampal synaptic plasticity and cognitive deficits induced by prenatal chronic stress. Neurobiol Learn Mem. 2007;87(2):257–63.
49. Champagne DL, Bagot RC, van Hasselt F, et al. Maternal care and hippocampal plasticity: evidence for experience-dependent structural plasticity, altered synaptic functioning, and differential responsiveness to glucocorticoids and stress. J Neurosci. 2008;28(23):6037–45.
50. van Hasselt FN, Cornelisse S, Yuan Zhang T, et al. Adult hippocampal glucocorticoid receptor expression and dentate synaptic plasticity correlate with maternal care received by individuals early in life. Hippocampus. 2012;22(2):255–66.
51. Wong-Goodrich SJ, Glenn MJ, Mellott TJ, Blusztajn JK, Meck WH, Williams CL. Spatial memory and hippocampal plasticity are differentially sensitive to the availability of choline in adulthood as a function of choline supply in utero. Brain Res. 27 2008;1237:153–66.
52. Wong-Goodrich SJ, Mellott TJ, Glenn MJ, Blusztajn JK, Williams CL. Prenatal choline supplementation attenuates neuropathological response to status epilepticus in the adult rat hippocampus. Neurobiol Dis. 2008;30(2):255–69.
53. Wong-Goodrich SJ, Tognoni CM, Mellott TJ, Glenn MJ, Blusztajn JK, Williams CL. Prenatal choline deficiency does not enhance hippocampal vulnerability after kainic acid-induced seizures in adulthood. Brain Res. 21 2011;1413:84–97.
54. West T, Atzeva M, Holtzman DM. Pomegranate polyphenols and resveratrol protect the neonatal brain against hypoxic-ischemic injury. Dev Neurosci. 2007;29(4–5):363–72.
55. Cysneiros RM, Ferrari D, Arida RM, et al. Qualitative analysis of hippocampal plastic changes in rats with epilepsy supplemented with oral omega-3 fatty acids. Epilepsy Behav. 2010;17(1):33–8.

# Contents

# Chapter 1
# Enhancing Childhood Development in a Normal Child

**Keywords** Normal development • Gross motor skills • Fine motor skills • Behavioral Skills • Stimulation • Developmental care • Early intervention • Mother child interaction

*The most important need for a child is to know that he is loved and cared for.*

Early childhood is the most intensive period of development where rapid brain growth is occurring; this affects cognitive, social, and emotional growth for the entire lifespan.

Adequate stimulation and nutrition in the first 3–5 years of life are essential for optimal development. Thus enhancing development helps ensure that each child reaches his or her own developmental potential. Who is better suited to enhance this development in the early ages other than the mother or the primary caregiver? Therefore optimizing this relationship between mother/caregiver and child is crucial, especially in the first 5 years of age.

In this chapter, we are proposing general tips as advice to the caregiver in order to help enhance early development in all its various aspects or domains.

D. Sinno et al., *Enhancing Early Child Development:*
*A Handbook for Clinicians*, DOI 10.1007/978-1-4614-4827-3_1,
© Springer Science+Business Media, LLC 2013

## Newborn

During this period newborns require their basic needs of nutrition, sleep, and daily care essentially met in order to survive. Beyond the survival, infants need nurturing, love, and attention. The advice to be given to mothers at this age can be summarized as follows:

- Breast-feed to give your baby breast milk 8–12 times per day to protect him from infections.
- Hold him, cuddle him, rock him, hug him.
- Talk to him, sing to him during bathing or feeding.
- Let him listen to soft music.

| *Fact* | *Avoid* | *Avoid* |
|---|---|---|
| Babies start learning at birth through seeing, hearing, feeling and moving | Wrapping the newborn tightly with a cloth (swaddling) for long periods of time – they should be able to move their limbs | Covering babies' faces for long periods of time to allow their eyesight to develop |

As infants grow they develop new skills; further stimulation builds on those skills to enhance them. The following section contains advice to mothers/caregivers on stimulation of specific domains of development.

## 1–3 Months

### In addition to previous activities
*For developing language skills and understanding:*

- Talk to your baby often; for example, say what you are doing: like dressing, bathing, feeding.

| *Fact* |
|---|
| Children at this age like to see faces and make new sounds |

- Make baby sounds (cooing sounds) while looking and smiling to your baby. Speak in a pleasant voice.
- Let your baby hear different sounds like music, rattles, squeaky noise from toys, etc.

> ### *Understand*
>
> *Copying the sounds and movements a child makes help the caregivers pay closer attention and understand the child easily*

*For developing personal and social skills:*

- When the baby cries, he is trying to communicate a need he has, so try to respond right away and comfort him.
- Talk to him in a soothing tone, rock him to relax.
- Show him books or toys with bright colors.
- Respond right away to him when he cries.
- Look at him when you talk to him and smile especially when he smiles back at you.
- Let him watch people and activities.

*For developing control of large muscles:*

- Place him on his tummy for few minutes each day. Put toys in front of him to encourage head lift and control.
- Encourage him to move body from side to side by moving toys in front of him.
- Put the baby sitting on your lap while holding his head to encourage head control.

*For developing control of small muscles and solving problems:*

- Let him feel different objects and textures by rubbing them against his hands.
- Let him follow a colorful toy in your hand.
- Make sure the baby has a quiet time to explore his own world, babble to himself, and play on his own.

> ### *Communicate*
>
> *Practice in communication helps prepare the child for talking later    .*

# 3–6 Months

**In addition to previous activities**
*For developing language skills and understanding:*

- Play "talking back and forth." First he makes a noise and you listen. Then you make the same noise and he listens.
- Encourage him to turn his head towards sounds.
- Tell him about a toy and show him how to use it. Talk to him in complete sentences.
- Read short stories, sing songs.
- Provide him some quiet time.

*For developing personal and social skills:*

- Show your baby that you are happy when he makes his first sounds and repeat them back.
- Hold him in front of a mirror and show him himself. Play "Peekaboo" with him.
- Hide a toy under a cloth so that he can look for it.
- Massage his body to relax.
- Make bath-time fun play, encourage him to splash or kick water. Never leave him alone near any water.

*For developing control of large muscles:*

- Put him on his back and let him reach toys hanging from the sides of his crib or park.
- Put him on his tummy and encourage him to raise his head and push up on the arms to watch what is happening in the world around.
- Try to get him to roll over from stomach to back and from back to stomach.
- Hold him upright from under the arms and allow his feet to touch the bed or your lap.
- Help him sit up alone. Put him in the corner of a couch while surrounded by pillows to prevent him from falling.

*For developing control of small muscles and solving problems:*

- Put a rattle or other safe toy into his hand and pull on it gently to encourage him to hold onto things.
- Put a toy or other object in his hand and see if he changes it to the other hand. Offer two objects, one for each hand, at the same time.
- Let him play with blocks; show him how to bang them.

# 6–9 Months

**In addition to previous activities**
*For developing language skills and understanding:*

- Get the baby books with bright colors and read to him daily.
- Talk to him a lot.
- Look at pictures in magazines, point and name them.
- Point and name body parts.
- Play with him clapping games: "Pat-a-Cake," "If you're happy and you know it clap your hands," etc.

*For developing personal and social skills:*

- Hug, cuddle him, play "Peekaboo," Soothe and calm him.
- Give him the chance to smell good things such as food, flowers, and spices.
- Help him learn why some things are not safe. For example, if he goes to the oven or heater, tell him it hurts ("Hot").

*For developing control of large muscles:*

- Help the baby to pull to stand, try to get baby to walk holding on furniture or your hands.
- Try to get him to bounce up and down.
- Put toys in front of him and encourage him to crawl.

> **Be Patient**
>
> *Children experiment through playing with objects: watching how they fall & how they make noise*

*For developing control of small muscles and solving problems:*

- Give the baby chance to pick food and feed himself.
- Help him drink from a cup.
- Let him play with floating toys while bathing.
- Show baby how to put things in boxes; let him play with safe containers.
- Encourage baby to hold a large crayon and scribble on a paper.

> **Fact**
>
> *Children recognize their names before they can say them*

> **Remember**
>
> *Children understand words before they learn how to say them. They are aware of expressions such as anger*

## 9–12 Months

### In addition to previous activities

*For developing language skills and understanding:*

- Make puppets out of gloves or socks and encourage communication with puppets, play games, invent stories.
- Teach him to say mama or dada.
- Sing baby songs to him.

> **Talk**
>
> *At this age, most children cannot speak yet, however they learn how to connect certain words to things around them.*

- Tell him the names of people and things such as animals, colors, and parts of the body.

*For developing personal and social skills:*

- Help the baby hold a cup and drink from it.
- Let him have meals with the family; have him sit nearby for a short time.
- Help him follow easy directions.
- Show him how to pull a toy.

| *Remember* |
| --- |
| *Children may become afraid when they lose sight of a familiar caregiver* |

| *Discover* |
| --- |
| *Children at this age enjoy hiding games – they like to discover where certain things disappear to* |

*For developing control of large muscles:*

- Let him sit up all by himself.
- Help him walk with support.
- Encourage him to reach toys by walking or crawling.
- Provide push or pull toys for him to play with.
- Get him to bend over and pick up a toy on the floor without holding on to anything.
- Sit with him on the floor and play ball together.

*For developing control of small muscles and solving problems:*

- Let him pick up a crayon using his thumb and a finger.
- Help him put objects into a container.
- Encourage him to play with bathtub toys.
- Give him a chance to feed himself.
- Show him how to put large blocks one on top of the other and bang them together.
- Let him play safely in the kitchen while you work there. Keep one low drawer filled with plastic containers, lids, spoons, and other safe objects for him to play with.

## 12–15 Months

**In addition to previous activities:**

*For developing language skills and understanding:*

- Teach the baby keywords: milk, water, bed. Encourage the baby to say the words back.
- Help the baby to name things by having him repeat after you.
- While bathing or dressing, teach him body parts.
- Encourage the baby to make "music" by hitting things together with a rhythm.

> *Remember*
>
> *At this age, children can understand words, begin to speak and follow simple directions*

*For developing personal and social skills:*

- Give him only one simple direction at a time. For example, bring the ball.
- Show him how to pull off his clothes and how to use a spoon to feed himself.
- Reward him when he does something good, praise him and say "thank you."
- Let the child play with a doll to feed and take care of.
- Take him out to places such as zoo, playground, and beach; take him on a walk with you.

> *Remember*
>
> *Children should be soothed when upset and their efforts should be praised*

*For developing control of large muscles:*

- Give him a toy to pull while he walks.
- Help him learn to crawl up and down steps safely.
- Show him how to take steps backward.
- Play hide-and-seek games.
- Show him how to catch and throw a large ball.

> *Encourage*
>
> *Children need encouragement when learning to walk, to play new games and to apply new skills*

*For developing control of small muscles and solving problems:*

- Help him build a tower with blocks, show him how, play with him.
- Show him how to put things into containers and how to get them out.

# 15–18 Months

**In addition to previous activities**
*For developing language skills and understanding:*

- Encourage the child to say what he wants. For example, Tell him how to say, "I want some milk please." Praise him for putting words together.
- When he points, tell him what he could say. If he points to the cat, say it is a cat.
- While looking at picture books and magazines, ask him to tell you what the story is about.
- Give him a toy telephone and play games calling "granny" or "daddy."
- Read to him out loud.

*For developing personal and social skills:*

- Hug and kiss him, and try to get him to hug and kiss you back.
- Let him help you with everyday activities. Let him take a spoon to the table or put dirty clothes in the basket.
- Teach him to take care of his teeth by helping him brush his teeth with water.
- Play hide-and-seek with him. At first make it easy and as he gets better make it harder to find you.
- Plan frequent outings with him to a playground, zoo, or park.

*For developing control of large muscles:*

- Let him play pouring and squeezing during bathing or swimming. Use plastic bowls and containers.
- Let child play on a rocking horse (be sure that the horse cannot be tipped over).
- Show him how to play on swings and climbing equipment.
- Encourage walking on tiptoes, backward, and up and down stairs.
- Take him to parks or places when he can run and play with a ball.

*For developing control of small muscles and solving problems:*

- Encourage playing with blocks, big pieces of puzzles, drawing with crayons, and finger painting.
- Show him how to blow soap bubbles. Talk about how the bubbles look and feel.
- Show child how to thread things (like large buttons) in a string.

## 18–24 Months

**In addition to previous activities**
*For developing language skills and understanding:*

- Read nursery rhymes, sing songs, and try to have the child sing with you.
- While talking use short sentences and read to your child every day.
- If you elect to have your child watch TV, choose quality programs and talk with him about what you both see. Limit watching to no more than 1/2 to 1 hour per day.
- Look at books and magazines together, get your child to tell you what is happening in the pictures.
- Talk about what happened today and what will happen tomorrow, especially before he goes to bed.
- Teach your child to follow directions by asking him to do things, e.g., "bring me the yellow shirt, please."
- Point at different objects and tell their colors.

*For developing personal and social skills:*

- Show your child that playing together is fun.
- Find a friend for him to play with. Encourage them to play together, e.g., "horse" or "hide-and-seek."
- Help your child put puzzles together or build towers with shoe boxes, for example.
- Encourage your child to use a spoon and a fork to feed himself and include him in family meals.
- Teach him how to button, zip, and snap using a book or old clothes.
- Play "Dress up" or "Telephone" with him.

- Let him play in front of a mirror.
- Whenever possible, offer the child choices: for example would you like a banana or an apple?

*For developing control of large muscles:*

- Encourage your child to run, play in water, kick, throw, and catch a large ball.
- Show your child how to jump up and down by holding his hands for a few jumps.
- Show him how to balance on one foot.
- Show your child how to swing, clap, and dance while enjoying music.

*For developing control of small muscles and solving problems:*

- Encourage your child to play with different shapes and sizes, e.g., cut holes of different sizes and shapes into the top of a shoe box. Give your child things to put through these holes.
- Buy or make "play clay" or dough and let your child pull, cut, and squeeze it into different shapes (Play dough recipe: 1 tbs oil + 1 cup water + 2 cups flour + 3/4 tsp salt).

# 2–3 Years

## In addition to previous activities
*For developing language skills and understanding:*

- Read stories daily. Sing songs together like "London Bridge," "Ring around the Rosie," "Twinkle twinkle," and "The wheels on the bus."
- Listen to your child and do not rush him even if what he says does not make sense.
- Help your child learn his first and last name. Help him learn the colors, names of animals, plants, and pieces of clothing.

> **Teach**
>
> *At this age, children can listen and understand the difference between right and wrong*

> **Fact**
>
> *At this age, children learn to name things, count and match colors, shapes and size*

- Tell stories about him based on real events or invent new stories.
- Write down the stories that he tells. Read them back to him.

> **Remember**
>
> *Children should be corrected gently when wrong*

*For developing personal and social skills:*

- Encourage your child to dress without any help from you.
- Let him help you around the house, e.g., ask him to pick up his clothes and toys.
- Allow your child to dress up in old adult clothes.

*For developing control of large muscles:*

- Show him how to bounce a large ball to you. Then bounce it back so that he or she can catch it.
- Encourage climbing, running, jumping, balancing, and playing ball.

> **Remember**
>
> *Looking at picture books and reading stories to children prepares them for reading later*

- Have him play "Follow the Leader" and crawl, tiptoes, and bunny hop under tables, around chairs, over pillows.
- Let your child learn to pedal a tricycle.

*For developing control of small muscles and solving problems:*

- Play matching game (matching colors or shapes).
- Show him how to take things apart and put them back together again.
- Encourage play with puzzles, blocks, and toys that nest.
- Give your child an empty egg carton to use for "pockets" and have him sort things such as different shapes and colors.
- Show him how to match pictures with real things such as making a picture of a ball with a real ball.
- Show him how to group things in one, twos, threes, and so on. Tell him how many there are and help him count them.

- Give him a set of large kindergarten blocks to play with.
- Show him how to draw shapes such as circles, line, and so on.
- Teach him how to describe how things feel. Show him what is soft, sticky, hard, rough, or furry.

# 4 Years

**In addition to previous activities**
*For developing language skills and understanding:*

- Let your child tell you the stories from his favorite books.
- Play listening and guessing games with him, e.g., make the sound of different animals and let him guess what each animal is.
- Encourage your child's questions, be patient and answer in simple words.

*For developing personal and social skills:*

- Let your child help make and serve snacks and meals.
- Take your child to the zoo, public library, children's museum, or/ and other places that have special events for children his age.

*For developing control of large muscles:*

- Let your child help you do things around the house.
- Make an obstacle course with boxes, chairs, and tables and let him find his way around all these things.
- Encourage dancing to rhythmic music and follow directions.

*For developing control of small muscles and solving problems:*

- Let your child use play dough.
- Let him tear or cut paper and paste these pieces onto another paper.
- Let your child pour liquid (water) into large cups.
- Use follow-the-dot outlines for letters and shapes.

# 5 Years

### In addition to previous activities

*For developing language skills and understanding:*

- Read daily and help your child read.
- Help him read the words on street signs and labels on containers.
- Teach him his family's name, his phone number, and his address.

*For developing personal and social skills:*

- Let your child have a friend over so they can play games together.
- Play guessing games with him. Pretend to do something and let him guess what you are doing. Make different expressions with your face and let him tell you what feelings he sees on your face.
- Teach him about the healthy foods.
- Show him how to answer the phone and make a call especially in case of an emergency.
- Encourage your child to care for himself and his family. Give him a chore he would be responsible for like picking dirty laundry.
- Help your child learn how to get along with others, share and "give-and-take."
- Make him choose his own clothes.

*For developing control of large muscles:*

- Let your child practice hopping, climbing, and skipping.
- Let your child learn to pedal a bicycle with training wheels.

*For developing control of small muscles and solving problems:*

- Let your child have a job to do in the house like setting the table at meal time.
- Help him practice drawing and printing letters and numbers.
- Encourage child to dress and undress alone.
- Teach child shoe lacing.

# Further Reading

1. Berk LE. Child development. 8th ed. Boston: Pearson/Allyn and Bacon; 2009.
2. Altmann TR. The wonder years. A bantam book. Elk Grove Village, IL: American Academy of Pediatrics; 2006.
3. Harstad EB, Barbaresi WJ. Disruptive behavior disorders. In: Voight RG, Macias MM, Myers SM, editors. Developmental and behavioral pediatrics. Elk Grove Village, IL: American Academy of Pediatrics; 2011. p. 349–58.

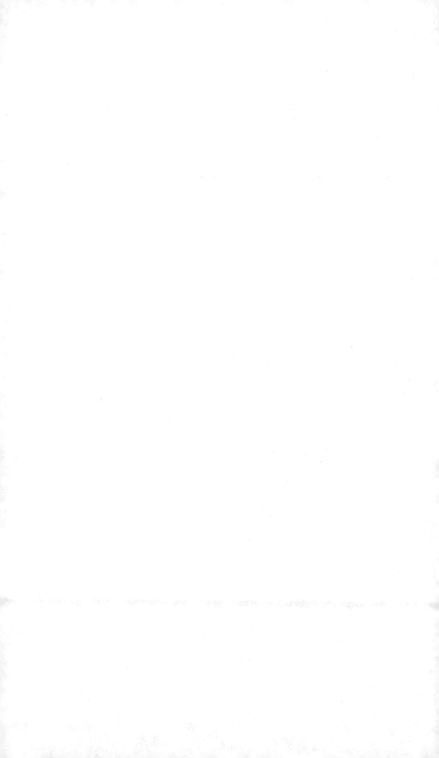

# Chapter 2
# Enhancing Childhood Development in Children with Autism

**Keywords** Autism • Asperger's syndrome • Speech delay • Early intervention • Pervasive developmental disorder • Autism • Interaction • Autism Communication

Autism spectrum disorder (ASD) refers to a group of neuro-developmental disorders that influence social interaction, communication, and cognitive development [1–3]. Autism is a spectrum disorder, with large variability in the presenting symptoms and their severity. Currently there is no cure for Autism or ASD; however, children diagnosed with ASD are capable of progressing developmentally and acquiring new skills in language and social interaction.

Early surveillance and screening for ASD is essential to ensure early detection and hence early referral for initiation of intervention programs and thus achieve a better outcome [1, 4].

According to the DSM-IV-TR, disorders such as "Asperger Syndrome," "Childhood Disintegrative Disease," "Rett's Disorder," and "Pervasive Developmental Disorder-Not Otherwise Specified" (PDD-NOS) are placed at one end of the spectrum, while others such as "Autism," "Classic Autism," and "Kanner Autism" are placed at the other end [5]. Children and adults with autism often show some intellectual disabilities [6].

D. Sinno et al., *Enhancing Early Child Development:*
*A Handbook for Clinicians*, DOI 10.1007/978-1-4614-4827-3_2,
© Springer Science+Business Media, LLC 2013

Manifestations of social and communication difficulties become clear before the age of 3 years [1–3, 6]. Issues in social development include unusual or delayed responses to social stimuli as well as low levels of social engagement and interest [1–3, 6, 7]. Additionally, autistic children exhibit problems and delays in language and self-care skills and often lack attention. Speech may be severely delayed or entirely absent in some cases of autism [1–3, 6, 7]. Routine behaviors and habits such as finger gazing, walking on toes, and hand gestures are noticeable among these children [1–3, 6, 7].

## Social Defects

Children with autism are sometimes withdrawn and comfortable with being alone and tend to avoid eye contact and attracting attention. They also exhibit difficulties in responding to gestures, vocalizations, and in emotional situations. They have problems in social interactions with other children through play and educational activities [1]. These social deficits and manifestations are often not clearly apparent at an early age and often overlooked, causing a delay in diagnosis of autism [1–3, 6, 7]. Table 1 outlines slight differences in social and behavioral development of children that may often be overlooked [1].

| Age | Typically developing children | Children with autism spectrum disorders |
|---|---|---|
| 10–12 months | Begin to follow a point | May not follow a point, even when one tries repeatedly to call their names in a loud voice or uses physical prompts |
| 12–14 months | Point to request an object | Make efforts by opening and closing their hand while it is raised in the direction of the desired item but without any back and forth looking between it and the caregiver |
| 14–16 months | Begin to point, to comment on or share an interesting object | Fail to point, to comment at age-appropriate times, and when they do, they are less likely to show positive affect and connectedness during the act |
| By 4 years of age | Begin to have some sense of other's mental state | Have difficulties with empathy, sharing, and comforting |
| *Novel situations* | Look to their mothers for an indication of delight, anger, or fear in facial expression. They may mimic hers, although they may not fully understand the situation | Engage in less imitation |

# Speech Deficits

Speech deficits may also be recognized at an early age given certain signs that may predict speech or language problems. Early on, the child lacks appropriate gaze in general and specifically does not exhibit expressions with his/her gaze. At approximately 6 months, the child vocalizes independently of his parents instead of mimicking the parents' vocalizations. Moreover, there is a general lack of response to and recognition of the primary caregiver's voice, even in cases where the child's name is called. At the age of 9 months, the child still exhibits a delay in babbling and using gestures such as waving or pointing. Moreover, the child does not use expressions or show interest in the expressions or statements of others [1].

# Communication with Autistic Children

A variety of interventions have been developed over the years for enhancing development and communication of children with autism [8]. For the purpose of this manual, the focus will be on enhancing communication with autistic children through daily activities that can be applied at home. Principles from "Daily Life Therapy" and the "Picture Exchange Communication System (PECS)" will be applied to improve communication, imitation, and self-care skills among these children [4, 9, 10].

## *Daily Life Therapy*

This therapy focuses on principles that encourage the establishment of a "rhythm" or routine in daily life [4, 10]. Its effectiveness lies in the fact that children with autism are often engaged in routine behaviors [1–3, 6, 7] and it builds upon that characteristic to teach them new skills.

For example, one can repeat certain words by putting it in simple sentences and encouraging the child to speak by asking him simple questions (Fig. 2.1).

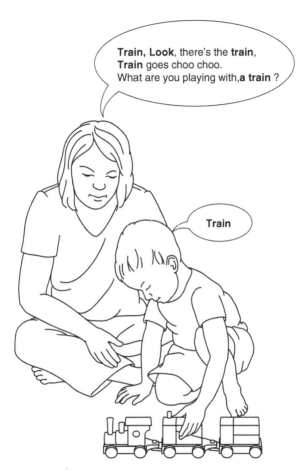

**Fig. 2.1** Mother encouraging child to speak by asking him simple questions

## *Picture Exchange Communication System*

PECS focuses on improving communication and language skills of children with autism within their social environments. It highlights the use of pictures as a communication technique to help them better visualize what they want or need [9] (Fig. 2.2).

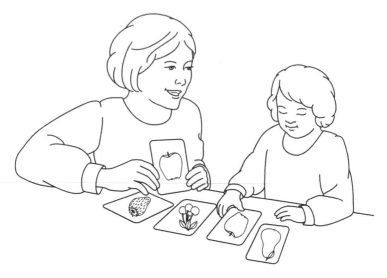

**Fig. 2.2** Use of pictures to communicate

## General Tips for Daily Activities

Following are advice the clinicians may give mothers and caregivers of children with autism in order to optimize various aspects of their development.

### Eating Tips

Encourage the child by inviting him to eat through singing (Fig. 2.3).

Encourage the child to communicate by speech. For example, prompt him to ask for more food by serving him with a small amount initially, forgetting to put a certain type so that he would notice it and ask for it (Fig. 2.4) or giving him the opposite of what he asked for to stimulate him to ask again for what he wants (Fig. 2.5).

Name the types of food by pointing at them, allow the child to point at the food that he wants (Fig. 2.6a). Show the child a list of two

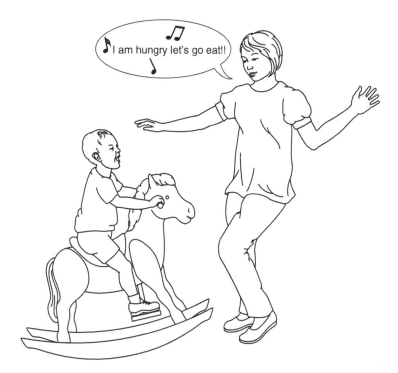

**Fig. 2.3** Tips to encourage eating

or three food choices and ask him to point out his choice. The list may be made up of pictures (Fig. 2.6b).

Repeat a certain sentence or song after every meal (Fig. 2.7).

## *Dressing Tips*

Encourage the child to participate in getting dressed by directing him to extend his arms or legs (Fig. 2.8). Accompany the actions with words and encourage him to repeat them (Fig. 2.9). Encourage the child to finish getting dressed on his own and praise him when he is done: "Good, you did it yourself" (Fig. 2.10). Accompany the child in choosing his clothes from the closet (Fig. 2.11). Arrange the child's clothes on the bed in an organized manner in order for him to choose his outfit (Fig. 2.12). Show the child pictures that explain the process

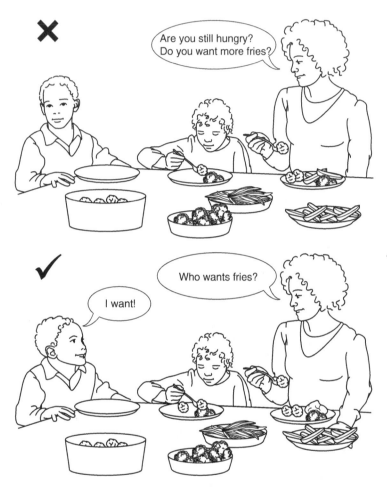

**Fig. 2.4** Tips to prompt child to communicate at the table

of getting dressed while giving him directions if possible (Fig. 2.13).

## Bathing Tips

Encourage the child to take a bath by singing or by pointing to things or repeating the same words every time (Fig. 2.14). Encourage the

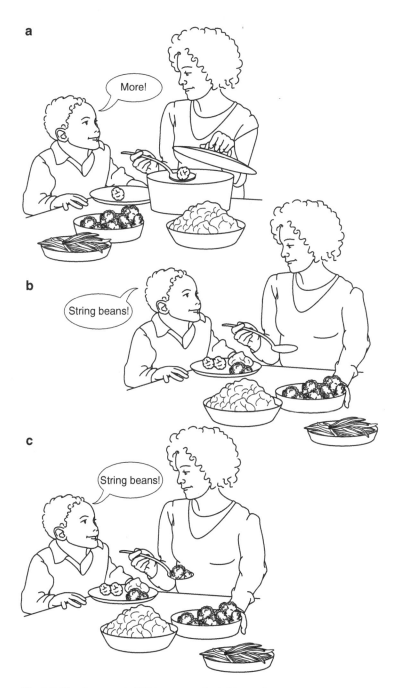

**Fig. 2.5** Tips to prompt child to communicate his needs

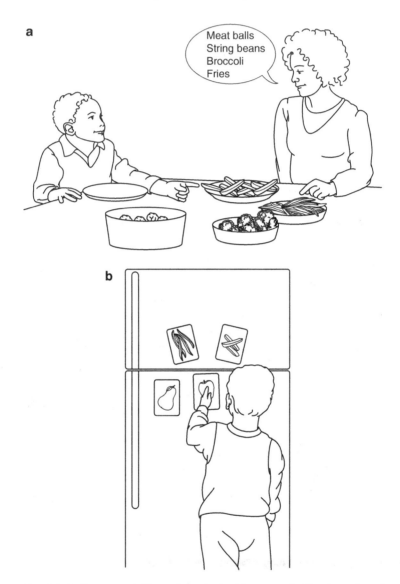

**Fig. 2.6** (a) Encourage child to point at the food he wants; (b) Use picture-list of different food items

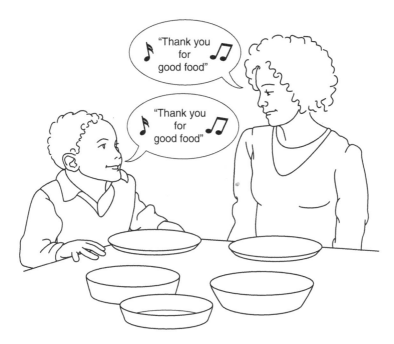

**Fig. 2.7** Communication through singing

child to participate in giving things (Fig. 2.15). Give the child toys that float or that can be filled with water to play with (Fig. 2.16). Teach the child about body organs and senses—repeat simple words slowly but in an expressive way (Fig. 2.17). Keep your position face to face with the child during bathing (Fig. 2.18). Allow the child to feel all the material to be used in bathing (Fig. 2.19). Show the child stages of bathing using pictures and/or words (Fig. 2.20). Repeat the same way of finishing the bathing each time. For example, put some calm music or repeat a certain song (Fig. 2.21).

## Entertainment

Entertainment is divided into four categories:

1. Social playing
2. Singing
3. Reading
4. Playing with toys

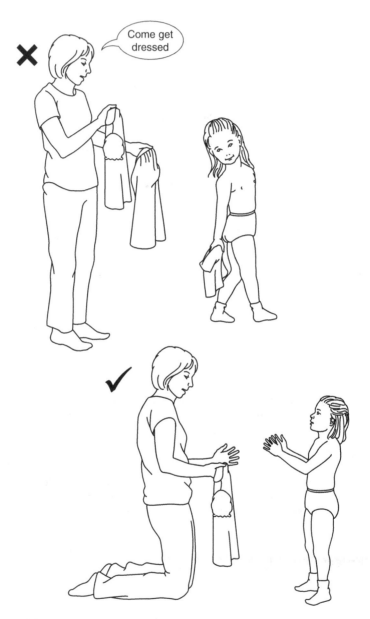

**Fig. 2.8** Tips for promoting child participation in getting dressed

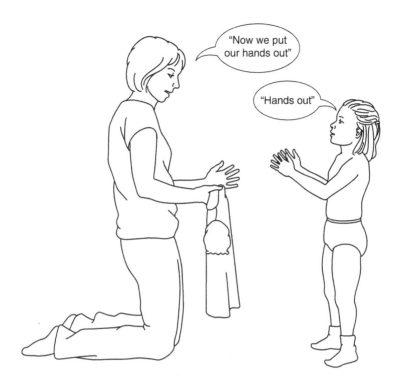

**Fig. 2.9** Dressing-up aid

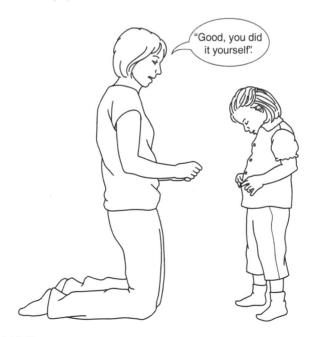

**Fig. 2.10** Tips to encourage autonomy

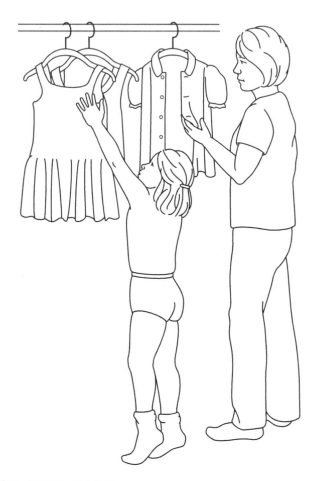

**Fig. 2.11** Choosing own cloth

## *Social playing*

This kind of playing requires from the child to communicate, to participate, and to react with others. It is organized and it is easy to predict what will happen. It involves feelings that relax the child: actions, words, and repetitive sounds. It is interesting and enjoyable. It can include: peekaboo, hide-and-seek, horse riding (on parent's leg) (Fig. 2.22), swinging, etc.

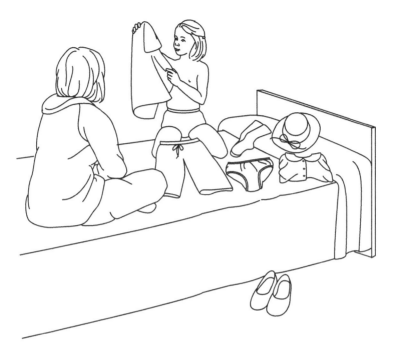

**Fig. 2.12** Arrange clothes on bed to help child choose his outfit

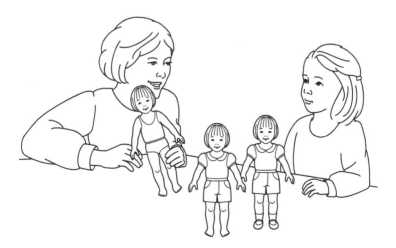

**Fig. 2.13** Use dolls to explain dressing process

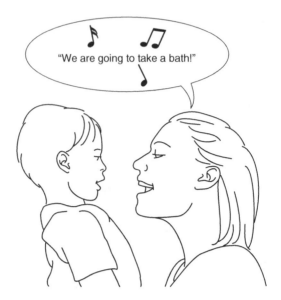

**Fig. 2.14** Tips to encourage taking a bath

a

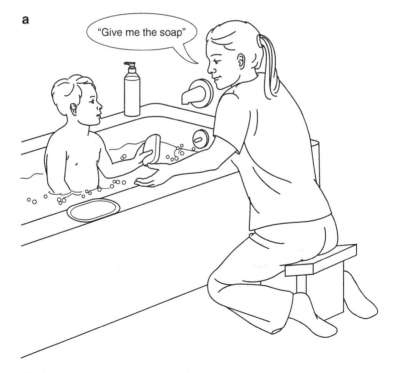

**Fig. 2.15** (a) Involve child in bathing process

b

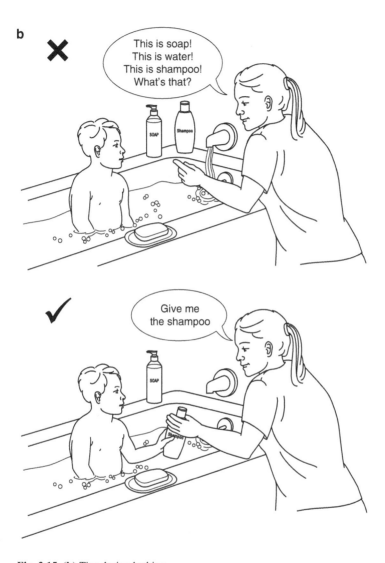

**Fig. 2.15** (**b**) Tips during bathing

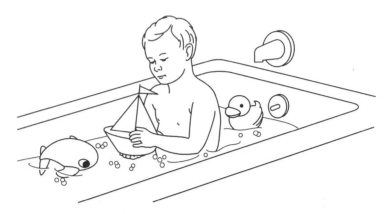

**Fig. 2.16** Make bath more enjoyable

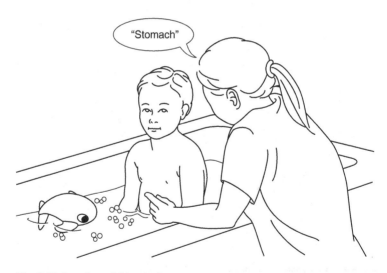

**Fig. 2.17** Introduce child to body parts

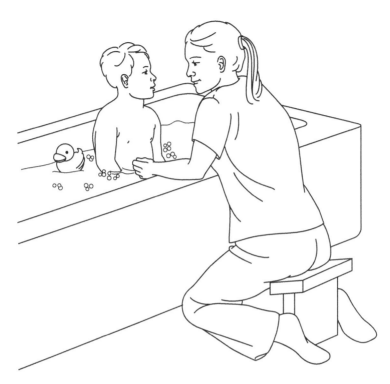

**Fig. 2.18** Interact with child during bath

**Preparation for the Activity**

Repeat what you say and do at the beginning of the activity, during, and at the end of the activity.

**During the Activity**

Give the child the opportunity to take roles (Fig. 2.23) and help him do this by getting involved in his interests and changing the way of play if necessary. For example, you are playing peekaboo with the child and you are hiding your face with a pillow and after some time of playing, the child goes to the curtains and hides behind them, you should continue the game by replacing the pillow with the curtains.

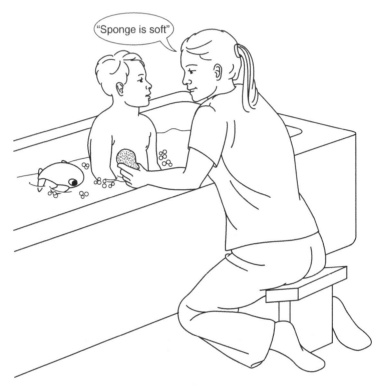

**Fig. 2.19** Make bathing environment familiar

## *Singing*

One can use songs to communicate with the child. The song is a way that we can repeat everyday so that the child will get used to it and memorize its words. We advise accompanying the song with suitable movements and pictures to make memorization easier (Fig. 2.24).

### During the Activity

- Give the child the opportunity to take roles.
- Stop on words and gestures he likes and encourage him to continue.

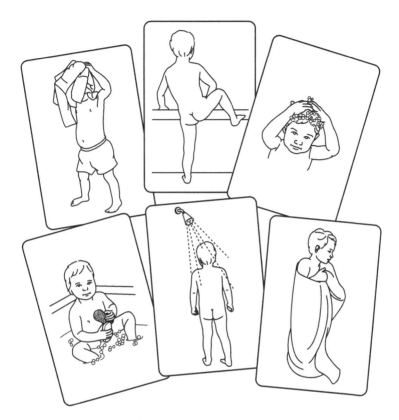

**Fig. 2.20** Teaching child the bathing process

- While singing, use few and simple words and stress on the main words.

One has to use or create songs especially for the child and that meet his needs in order to help him ask for things, ask questions then answer, greet others, understand daily routine, and simple guidelines.

## *Reading*

Reading is another way to strengthen communication with the child within enjoyable times that encourage interaction. As in songs, one has to repeat the same story several times.

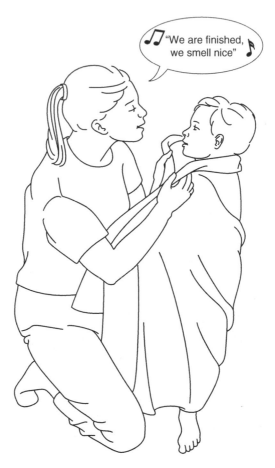

**Fig. 2.21** Finish bath with a song

**Reading the Right way**

- Read the story in an enjoyable and exciting manner to draw his attention.
- Stress on what interests him.
  - For example, if he points to a certain detail, one has to read the story while stressing this detail. [This is a way to communicate and to give information about what interests him.]

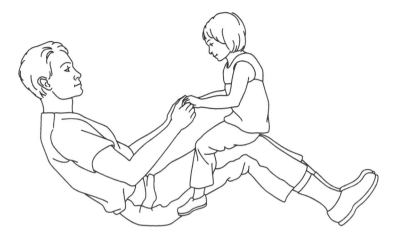

**Fig. 2.22** Promoting social interaction

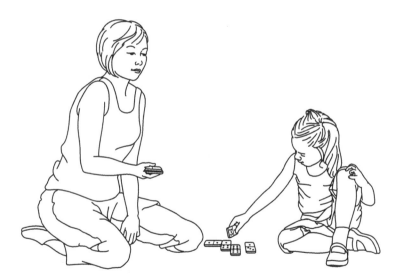

**Fig. 2.23** Playing and taking roles

- Simplify sentences.
  - It is advisable not to read in a traditional way but rather to simplify sentences so that it would suit the child's abilities.
- Read for him in a lively and expressive manner.

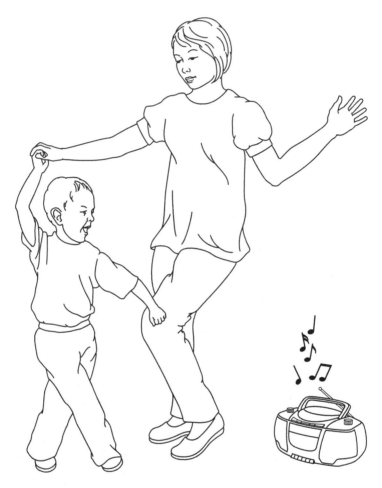

**Fig. 2.24** Promoting communication through songs

- If he wants to turn the pages, one has to participate with him doing this so that each one would turn one page of the book.
- Read slowly and repeat things.

  - One has to stress certain words by showing the corresponding pictures so that the child would understand, memorize, and use them in a spontaneous manner.
  - Give the child the opportunity to express his interests, one should not forget watching, slowing down, and explaining.

## *Playing with Toys*

Playing with toys is the easiest way to communicate with a child. One has to choose suitable toys such as visual environmental toys; toys with cause and result, sharing toys, building toys, blowing toys, toys with rules, symbolic toys, and physical play (Figs. 2.25 and 2.26).

### Playing Stage

- Ask the child to choose between two or more toys.
- Give him the toy he chose and watch him at a first stage without directing him.
- Imitate the way he plays and share with him his way of playing.

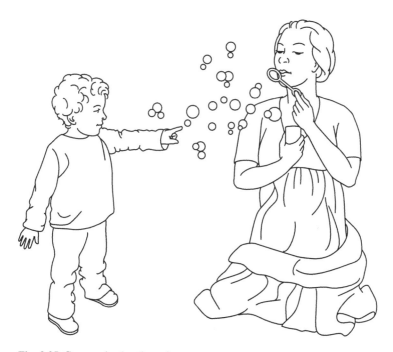

**Fig. 2.25** Communicating through toys

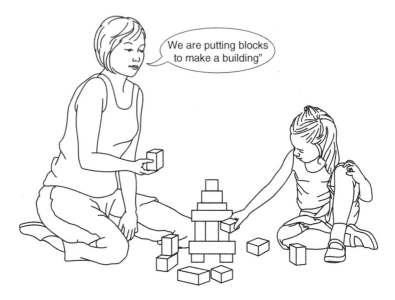

**Fig. 2.26** Parent playing with her child stating out loud what they are doing

- If he feels bored, one should continue playing before moving to another play.

Continuation is maintained by creating a new method of play and encouraging him to follow it.

- Take advantage of play time to enrich his language by simplifying words and sentences, stressing the main words, slowing down while talking, and pointing to what you are saying (Fig. 2.27).
- Finish the play in a routine way by a song for example (Fig. 2.28).

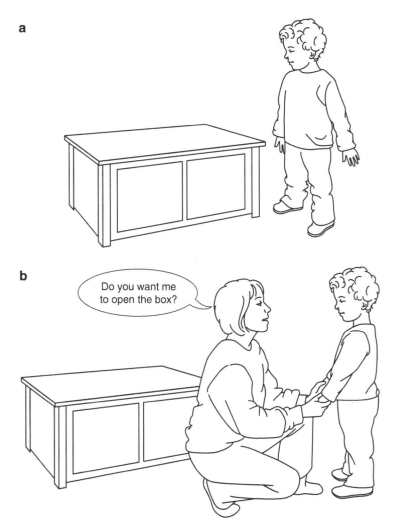

**Fig. 2.27** Parent encouraging child to play, (**a**) child looking not knowing what to do, (**b**) Parent inviting child by asking

## Daily Activities

The daily activities shown through a series of pictures have the potential to decrease the child's anxiety (Fig. 2.29).

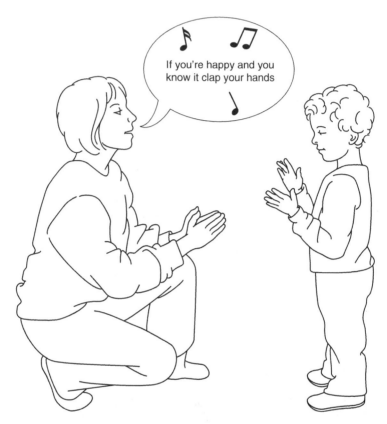

**Fig. 2.28** Parent finishing an activity with a song

## *How Does a Child with Autism Play?*

Playing is not easy for the child with autism. One can notice that he plays differently from what is expected since he chooses methods that suit him. The different ways used by those children depend on their way of communication with others and with the environment.

A child with autism:

1. Does not play with toys, rather he is interested in chewing them.
2. Plays in an unusual way not the way expected from a child his age.

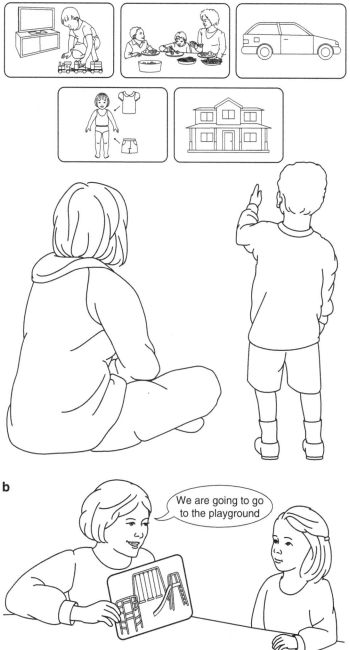

**Fig. 2.29** To decrease child's anxiety parent can use (**a**) a series of pictures or (**b**) one picture to explain what they are about to do

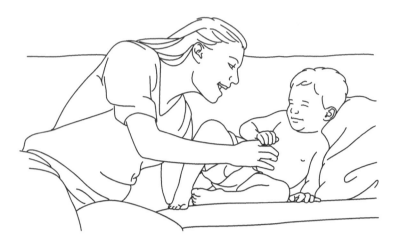

**Fig. 2.30** Parent eliciting a child reaction by tickling

3. Plays in a particular way: he can play the right way with some games such as puzzles; he has his favorite games but cannot generalize the right way of playing to different games, and he can perform one task only in the game.
4. Can play in a well-built manner: he can specify a goal and work to achieve it. He can use toys to do something (e.g., pencils and papers for drawing). Children with limited communication skills should be able to participate in such activities.
5. Can play games with rules: he can take roles and play with others in a limited way. Children with limited communication skills like repeating the same playing method over and over.
6. Can play symbolic and imaginary games: Symbolic playing is pretending to do something imaginary such as drinking from an empty cup. All children with autism except those who do not communicate with others at all are capable of playing symbolic and imaginary games but in different ways.

## *How to Play with a Child with Autism*

Playing with a child who has autism should go through the following stages:

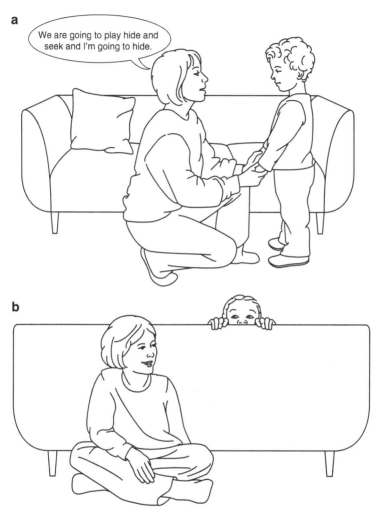

**Fig. 2.31** (**a**) Parent telling the child What they are doing. (**b**) Parent hiding from child

1. Joining the child's interests: Paying attention to the way the child plays and joining him.
2. Explaining the child's words and actions: Dealing with everything that the child does as if it is directed to us to build a connection with him through playing.

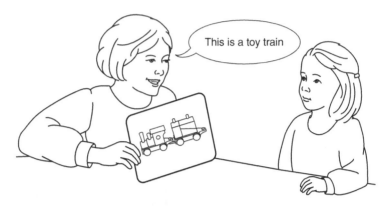

**Fig. 2.32** Parent showing a picture and naming the object

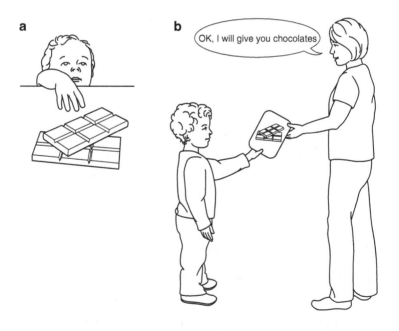

**Fig. 2.33** (**a**) Child unable to reach chocolate on the table. (**b**) Child giving parent a picture of chocolate to express his need

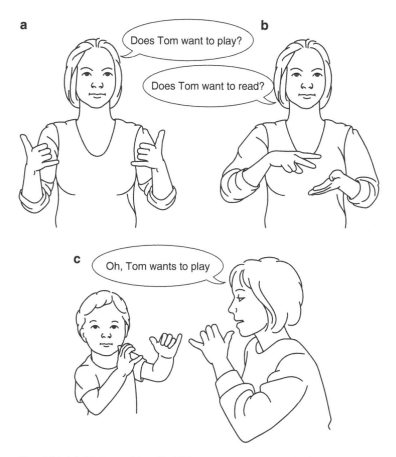

**Fig. 2.34** (**a**) Mother asking if child wants to play using hand gestures. (**b**) Mother asking if child wants to read. (**c**) Child repeating the sign to express his needs and mother confirming her understanding

3. Imitating the child: Imitating the way the child plays helps him to interact with us and encourages him to imitate us. The goal is to transform single playing into interaction and participation. There should be insistence in order to reach this goal because the child will not be responsive from the first time.
4. Entering into the child's world: Joining the child's play and insisting on that even if the child does not accept at first.
5. Repeating what we do and say: When we start playing, we should repeat the game's name and this would create a routine that the

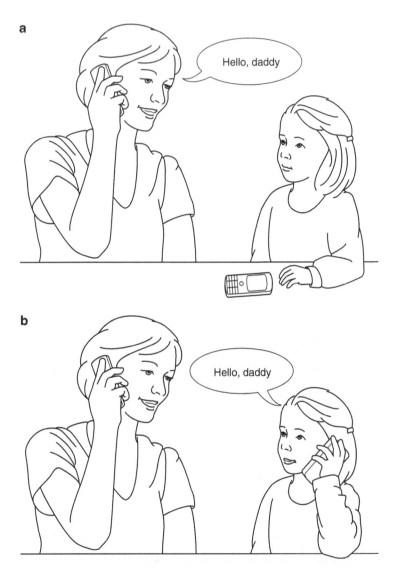

**Fig. 2.35** Mother helping child mimic answering the phone

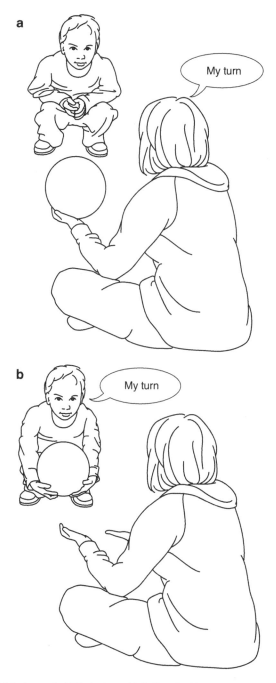

**Fig. 2.36** Mother and child playing with ball and taking turns

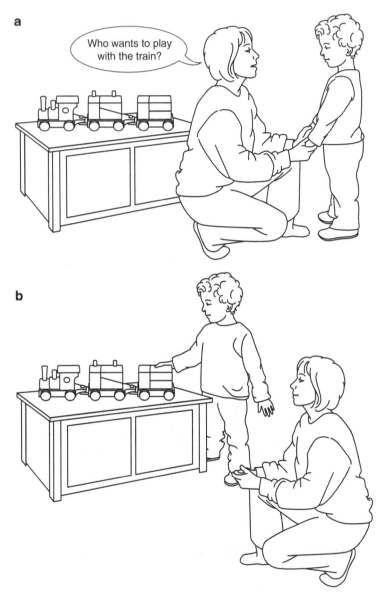

**Fig. 2.37** Mother plays and direct her child's play encouraging him to talk

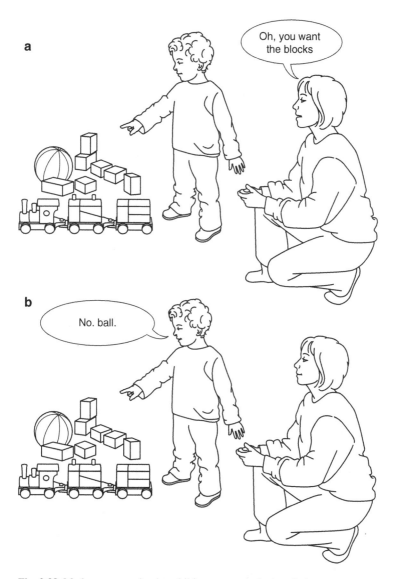

**Fig. 2.38** Mother encouraging her child to name toys he is pointing at

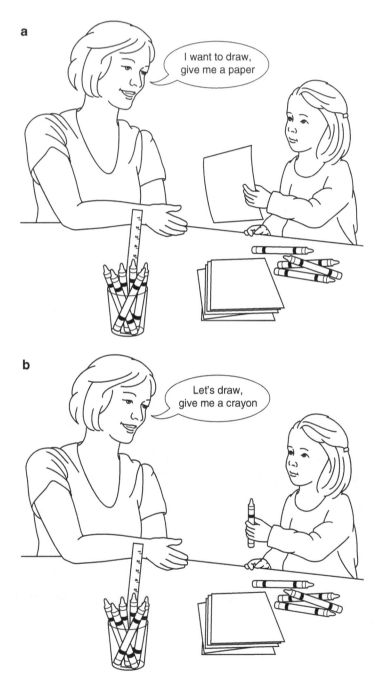

**Fig. 2.39** Mother encouraging child to follow commands and be an active player

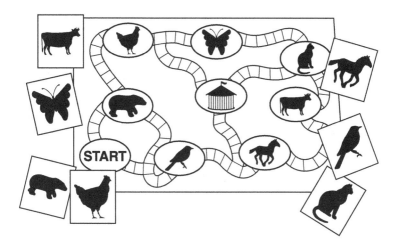

**Fig. 2.40** Board games involving matching pictures are helpful for playing together

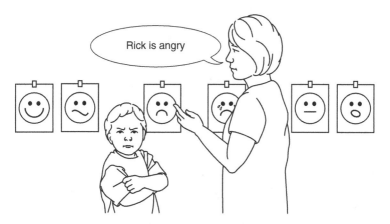

**Fig. 2.41** Mother alternating pictures displaying emotions

child gets used to and pushes him to expect what will happen. During playing, should applaud for him after each stage or count 1, 2, 3 before each stage of the play. To help the child generalize what he learned with us, one should repeat the game and the way used with other people.

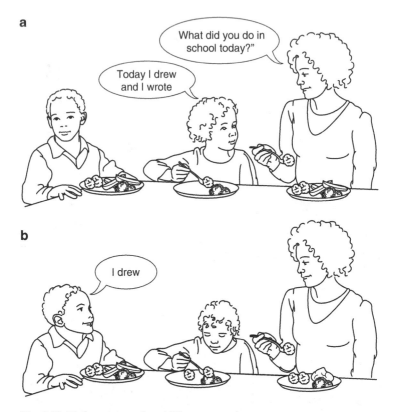

**Fig. 2.42** Mother encouraging child to communicate

6. Giving the child a chance to take roles: Planning for specified times to make the child take roles which means one should not continue playing but should stop to give the child the opportunity to take the initiative in specified times. Planning for a role for we want the child to take which means organizing the game in such a way to allow the child to participate in it.
7. Pointing to the child to help him take roles in the first stage: The child will not take his role in a spontaneous way. One should help him by giving clear signs. These signs could be body hints, body and verbal examples, or verbal instructions.
8. Continuing the enjoyable activity: the child with autism gets bored easily and does not concentrate for a long time. Thus, one has to revive the game and continue with it as much as possible.

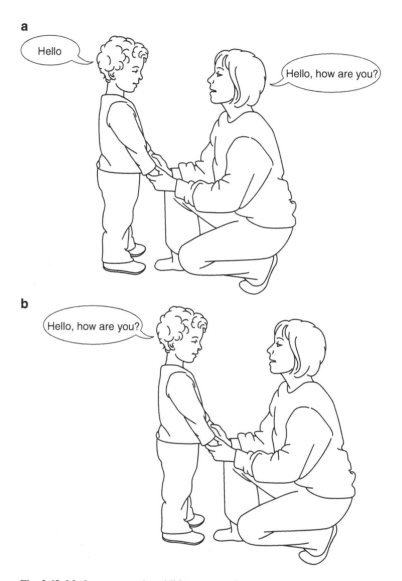

**Fig. 2.43** Mother encouraging child to communicate

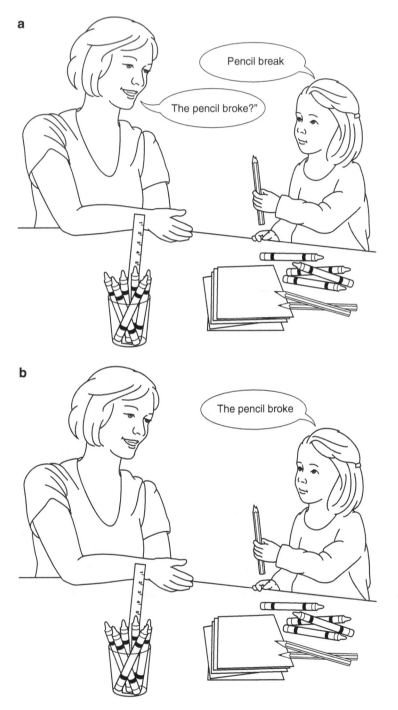

**Fig. 2.44** Child showing his broken pencil trying to communicate

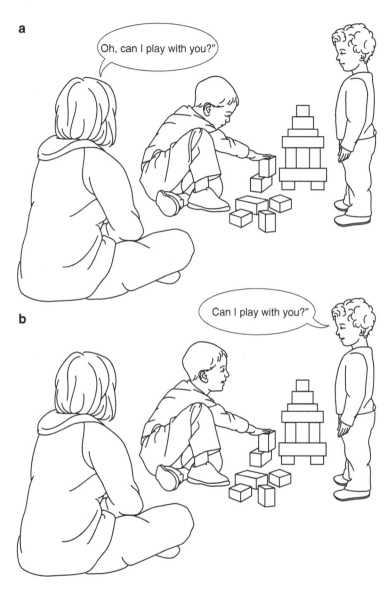

**Fig. 2.45** Mother and child playing with toys

**Types of toys a child with autism can play with**

1. Toys with cause and result: these toys are the easiest because all autistic children are able to play with them whatever their method is. It is enough for the child to press on a button or open a box to hear a sound or to see something in front of him.
2. Visual environmental toys: These toys require recognizing easy shapes. It is enough for the child to look at them in order to understand them.
3. Building toys: These toys allow the child to build the shapes he wants.
4. Sharing toys: such as balls and keys. These toys encourage the child to share playing through giving toys to us then taking them back. The child will consider us as part of the game.
5. Blowing and music toys: These are easy toys and the best to teach the child how to play. They include balloons, soap blowing and music boxes. The goal is to create communication and interaction with the child. Through this play process one has to create difficulties the child cannot overcome on his own. This pushes him to ask for help to blow soap balloons for example.
6. Creativity playing: This type of playing stimulates children because it helps them experience new feelings. These include playing with sand, water, cotton, rice, papers, board, coloring pencils...
7. Symbolic games: These are the toys that resemble real things such as cars and phones. They stimulate the child to do things similar to real life.
8. Physical playing: These games require physical activity and interaction with other children. These include swings, bicycles, wood horses...
9. Games with rules: These are board games with rules found inside the box in general. To play with those games at least two people are required to follow the rules. However, rules can be simplified or new rules can be created to match the child's level of understanding.

## Four Ways of Life for a Child with Autism

| 1 | 2 | 3 | 4 |
|---|---|---|---|
| The child who lives in his own world | The child who asks for others | The child who communicates in a primitive way | The child who communicates with us |
| 1. Does not interact with his environment. <br> 2. Does not understand yet that he can affect other people in his environment through sending a verbal or nonverbal message. <br> 3. Despite the lack of communication, his body language can translate and explain his feeling. | 1. Understands that his actions can affect his environment. <br> 2. Takes other people's presence into consideration and asks for help. | 1. Can interact in certain encouraging and enjoyable situations and ask for things important for him (such as his favorite toy or food). <br> 2. Communicates with purpose however in a limited way, i.e., limited to asking others to do what he wants. <br> 3. Can understand only simple and short sentences directed to him. | 1. Can interact with people and use verbal language for communication. <br> 2. Has no understanding of the communication rules especially in strange situations. <br> 3. Relies on repeating other people's words or sentences when he cannot express himself in his own way. |

## Communication with the *child who lives in his own world*

This child does not interact with his environment because he has not understood yet that he can affect other people in his environment through sending a verbal or nonverbal message.

*Draw the child's attention and push him to interact with you through social playing (Fig. 2.26)*

Make games interesting and encouraging: Draw his attention by tickling him, then putting him on your lap to play riding the horse. Join the child when he is playing alone. Call him to play a certain game by naming it with an encouraging rhythm and voice.

Repeat the same games so that the child would get used to them and learn them. This way we can encourage the child to interact with the game.

Explain everything that the child does unintentionally as a sign to communicate with you. If you were interested in all his actions and your reaction was positive, the child will be encouraged to repeat these actions.

*Create situations to push the child to communicate (Fig. 2.27)*

Keeping away or hiding the thing that the child wants.

Close the toy box to stimulate him to ask for opening it.

*Stimulate the child to take roles through body signs, eye contact, easy songs, or when he badly wants something (Fig. 2.28)*

Give the child body signs to take his role.

Help him physically to interact with you.

Give him an example to imitate.

Wait for the child and look at him to take his role.

Slow the game down.

*Help the child understand words and expressions as much as possible (Fig. 2.29)*

Name things, people, actions, and situations so that he would start linking words to things. This way the child has an example to imitate.

Show him examples of pictures of things you are talking about.

Use the name of the child when talking to him instead of saying "you"—this draws his attention and helps him learn his name.

Use funny and interesting words. The child likes these words and learns them easily.

Accompany what you say with signs and facial expressions to help him understand the words used.

*Diversify the games you play with the child: types of games include peekaboo, tickling, hide-and-seek, and the horse game (Fig. 2.30)*

Choose the toys in a suitable way: toys with cause and result, visual and environmental toys, building toys, sharing toys, creativity toys, symbolic toys, and physical games.

Show the child that the game is interesting even if he is playing it wrong. It is more important for him to enjoy the game than to play it correctly.

Help the child learn how to play simple games. Give him the opportunity to play in his own way and encourage him when he does something correctly.

Help the child interact through sharing games such as the ball game.

Imitate what the child does to draw his attention and continue the interaction.

*\* If we had a plan for certain game and the child started to play in a different way, we should follow the child and his interests*

*\*Do not forget to talk to the child slowly and clearly*

### Communication with *the child who asks for others*

This child can understand that his actions can affect his environment. He takes our presence into consideration and asks for our help.

*Encourage the child to use new ways to ask for physical games such as tickling or hide-and-seek (Fig. 2.31)*

When the child gets used to a game, you can change it or change the way you play it by making mistakes on purpose. Create a routine that the child gets used to, then change it suddenly. Hide things in unusual places. Surprise him with touch and smell senses.

Change the way the child asks to participate in a certain physical game.

Help him communicate for new reasons (different from requests) within the usual games: Give him choices between different ways to take roles. Follow his interests when he takes a certain initiative. If the child does not like to change the way of playing, do not give up and wait for him to accept the change—do not force the change.

Help the child use the roles learned during games, songs, books, or activities. Help the child generalize. Some of the activities that encourage the child to communicate are the peekaboo and hide-and-seek games.

*Help the child develop or change his body communication (Fig. 2.32)*

Encourage him to use signs, pictures, sounds, or words.

Put pictures next to the things they represent or in a small booklet to help him use them.

Repeat signs and words according to the level of the child and play guessing games with him.

*Increase the situations that give the child the chance to ask for new things (Fig. 2.33)*

Put things he likes in places that cannot be reached.

Give him what he wants step by step.

Give him what he wants except for one thing.

*Help the child understand words and expressions as much as possible (Fig. 2.34)*

*Same as this section in communication with the first type*

*Diversify the games you play with the child (Fig. 2.35)*

The games suggested in communication with the first type can be used.

Play differently within the same game.

Encourage the child to imitate you during symbolic playing such as talking over the phone.

Help him respond to your requests and directions. For example, put the apple in the plate.

*Encourage the child to generalize playing with other people such as the grandparents and siblings. This way he is encouraged to generalize what he learned by using the same way with other people from his environment.*

**Communication with the *child who communicates in a primitive way***

This child can interact in certain enjoyable and encouraging situations and ask for things important for him (such as his favorite toy or food). He communicates on purpose but this communication remains limited to asking others to do what he wants. He can understand words directed to him if we use simple and short sentences.

*The child learns to take roles regularly with physical playing (Fig. 2.36)*

Give the child a verbal example about the expressions that he can use of words or simple sentences. This allows him to use these words and pictures through imitating and repeating what he hears.

Give him signs so that he can understand that he has to repeat the example he is seeing or continue the expression we started with.

Start with a sentence that he has to continue.

Ask questions such as: open questions with choices, closed questions that can be answered by yes or no, questions that start with who or what.

*Encourage the child to take the initiative with physical playing instead of waiting for you to start the game (Fig. 2.37)*

Give him signs that help him take the initiative.

Develop signs to reach communication by pictures.

Develop communication by pictures to reach verbal communication.

Develop words to reach sentences.

*Encourage him to help communicate in different situations (Fig. 2.38)*

Refuse and protest.

Use greeting expressions.

Draw your attention to a person or a thing.

Comment on an unusual thing.

*Help the child understand words and sentences as much as possible and follow simple directions (Fig. 2.39)*

Use correct and simple sentences to help him hear the spoken language rules and use them later on.

Name things, people, actions and situations the right way.

Use the names of people after using pronouns.

Help him understand that every word in the sentence has its own meaning and that words have connection in between them within the sentence.

*Diversify the games that you play with the child (Fig. 2.40)*

Beside the games proposed in the first and second ways, symbolic games and games that have specific rules can be used.

## Communication with the *child who communicates with us*

This child can interact with us and use verbal language as a way of communication, but he has not understood yet all the rules of communication especially in strange situations. He relies on repeating words or sentences when he cannot express using his own way.

*Help the child change his way of communication (Fig. 2.41)*

Exchange repeated words by special words for the child. When his ability to understand gets better, repeating the same words regresses.

Use correct words and sentences during speech.

Use pictures for subjects that the child cannot express verbally such as feelings.

*Help him communicate: The child can comment on what he sees, draw attention by calling or answering. Get him to apply what he learned with you or other people and in new situations. Help him communicate & talk about hypothetical situations (Fig. 2.42)*

Encourage him to answer questions that start with "what, who, where, why, how". Use questions in simple songs, so he can get used to asking them.

Show him pictures that have the answers and ask him to choose.

Benefit from physical games such as hide-and-seek by repeating questions like "where are you?"

The questions that start with "why" and "how" are the most difficult. Make the questions understandable by giving him the answer and expect from him yes or no.

Talk about the past and the future, about feelings.

Play acting games with the roles of mother and father.

*Help the child make a conversation by teaching him (Fig. 2.43)*

How to start and end a conversation.

How to stick to the conversation's subject.

To understand that people do not always understand what he says and he has, in this case, to change the way he addresses others.

To ask others to clarify what they are saying.

To respect the conversation rules within social playing.

*Help him develop his ability to understand speech (Fig. 2.44)*

Break down long sentences.

Stress on abstract words by accompanying them with signs & repeating them in different sentences.

If you notice that the child does not understand the words addressed to him because he repeats what was said without changing anything in the sentence, you can simplify the sentence to make it understandable.

Repeat what the child says in a right way to correct the mistakes he committed without asking him to repeat what he said.

While talking with child, address abstract issues such as how he behaves and how to overcome obstacles.

*Help him communicate in an effective way with other children (Fig. 2.45)*

Teach the child how to start a game with another child.

Teach the child how to stay within the game, so that he can respect its rules with other children. Later, he can generalize it with others.

Teach the child how to end the game by using certain expressions.

# References

1. Johnson CP, Myers SM, The Council on Children with Disabilities. Identification and evaluation of children with autism spectrum disorders. Pediatrics. 2007;120(5):1183–215.
2. Rapin I, Tuchman RF. Autism: definition, neurobiology, screening, diagnosis. Pediatr Clin North Am. 2008;5:1129–46.
3. Volkmar F, Chawarska K, Klin A. Autism in infancy and early childhood. Annu Rev Psychol. 2005;56:315–36.
4. Warren Z, McPheeters ML, Sathe N, Foss-Feig JH, Glasser A, Veenstra-Vanderweele J. A systematic review of early intensive intervention for autism spectrum disorders. Pediatrics. 2011;127(5).
5. American Psychiatric Association. Diagnostic and statistical manual of mental disorders, text revision (DSM-IV-TR). 4th ed. Washington: American Psychiatric Publishing; 2000.
6. Kanner L. Autistic disturbances of affective contact. Nerv Child. 1943;2:217–50.
7. Volkmar FR, Chawarska K. Autism in infants: an update. World Psychiatry. 2008;7:19–21.
8. Heflin LJ, Simpson RL. Interventions for children and youth with autism: prudent choices in a world of exaggerated claims and empty promises. Part I: Intervention and treatment option review. Focus Autism Other Dev Disabl. 1998;13(4):194–211.
9. Bondy A, Frost L. The picture exchange communication system. Behav Modif. 2001;25(5):725–44. Review Larkin AS and Gurry S (1998) Brief report: progress reported in three children with autism using daily life therapy. J Autism Dev Disord. 28(4):339–42.
10. Quill K, Gurry S, Larkin A. Daily life therapy: a Japanese model for educating children with autism. J Autism Dev Disord. 1989;19(4):625–35.

# Chapter 3
# Enhancing Childhood Development in Children with Cerebral Palsy and Other Disorders

**Keywords** Cerebral palsy • Early intervention • Motor disability • Ataxia • Spasticity • Dystonia • Physical positioning

## Introduction

Infants and children who manifest motor dysfunction early in life have decreased ability to interact with their environment which results in less learning opportunities; hence, the consequent cognitive impairment often seen in these circumstances. During this period of brain growth, the brain plasticity allows the rewiring and the creation of new synapses that would compensate for the motor and cognitive deficits [1]. Therefore, early intervention to limit the physical disability and encourage motility, especially before the age of three has the potential to increase the chances of limiting or overcoming further developmental disabilities and promoting alternative learning methods to accomplish challenging tasks.

Studies looking at benefits of early intervention in cases of cerebral palsy have shown improved motor outcome correlating with the number of interventions [2–6].

D. Sinno et al., *Enhancing Early Child Development: A Handbook for Clinicians*, DOI 10.1007/978-1-4614-4827-3_3, © Springer Science+Business Media, LLC 2013

# Cerebral Palsy

The term cerebral palsy (CP) means literally "brain *paralysis*" or weakness [7]. CP is the most common physical disability in childhood affecting 2–3/1,000 live births in Western countries, with a higher incidence in premature and twin births [2, 3, 8].

## *What Is CP and What Causes It?*

- CP is an "**umbrella**" or a basket of terms covering nonprogressive but changing impairments that affect movement, balance, and posture. These conditions often result from lesions or anomalies affecting the brain in its early stages of development [2, 9].
- The new definition submitted to *Developmental Medicine and Child Neurology in 2006* [8] can be summarized as follows:

  - "Cerebral palsy describes a group of permanent disabilities or disorders in movement and posture development causing limitations in activity and body deformities.
  - These disabilities are attributed to nonprogressive disturbances that occurred during brain development in the fetus or infant.
  - The motor disorder or disabilities are often accompanied by comorbidities including epilepsy, learning difficulties, behavioral challenges, and sensory impairments in addition to secondary musculoskeletal problems [2, 8, 9]".

- CP is a lifelong condition which symptoms range from mild to severe but do not get worse with age; most children improve significantly with treatment [8, 9].
- Etiologies and risk factors include: [2, 3, 8, 10]

  - Infections during pregnancy
  - Maternal iodine deficiency
  - Blood clotting disorders in mother or infant
  - Inflammation
  - Prematurity
  - Twin gestation
  - Perinatal asphyxia
  - Brain malformations
  - Severe jaundice or Kernicterus
  - Genetic conditions

# *When to Suspect CP?*

Cerebral palsy should be suspected whenever a child shows differences in motor development as asymmetric function or unusual **muscle stiffness or floppiness**. Identification of these abnormal motor posture and function can be made **at 6 months of age or sooner** [4, 8]. Usually children with CP fail to reach their normal motor milestones in the first 12–18 months of age [2].

* CP should be suspected if [11]:

  – A 2 months or older child has difficulty controlling her head or has stiff legs that cross or "scissor" when picked up
  – A 6 months or older child reaches with only one hand while keeping the other in a fist
  – A 10 months or older child crawls by pushing off with one hand and leg while dragging the opposite hand and leg
  – A 12 months or older child **cannot crawl nor stand with support**

**Description of Cerebral Palsy**

CP is usually described by topography, functional status, and type.

1. Topography [2, 12] (Fig. 3.1):

   * Hemiparesis or hemiplegia: unilateral impairment of arm or leg on the same side
   * Diplegia: motor impairment primarily of legs (some involvements of arms)
   * Triplegia: three limb involvement
   * Quadriplegia (tetraplegia): all four limbs are functionally compromised

2. Functional status or severity of CP: gross motor function classification system (GMFCS) [13, 14] (Table 3.1 and 3.2)

Types of Cerebral Palsy

*Spastic Cerebral Palsy*

The Centers for Disease Control and Prevention estimate that around 70–80 % of children with cerebral palsy are spastic [15]. Spasticity refers to an **uncontrollable increase in the muscle tension** of the

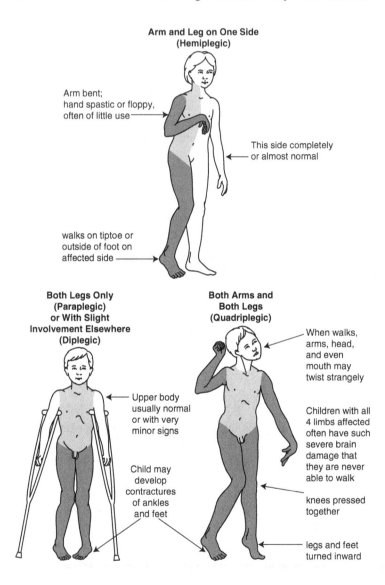

**Fig. 3.1** Topography of Cerebral Palsy

**Table 3.1** GMFCS of children less than 2 years

| Level I | • Move in and out of sitting and floor sit with both hands free to manipulate objects. |
|---|---|
| | • Crawl on hands and knees, pull to stand and take steps holding on to furniture. |
| | • Walk between 18 months and 2 years of age without the need for any assistive mobility device. |
| Level II | • Maintain floor sitting but may need to use their hands for support to maintain balance. |
| | • Creep on their stomach or crawl on hands and knees. |
| | • May pull to stand and take steps holding on to furniture. |
| Level III | • Maintain floor sitting when the low back is supported. |
| | • Roll and creep forward on their stomachs. |
| Level IV | • Have head control but trunk support is required for floor sitting. |
| | • Can roll to supine and may roll to prone. |
| Level V | • Physical impairments limit voluntary control of movement. |
| | • Unable to maintain antigravity head and trunk postures in prone and sitting. |
| | • Require adult assistance to roll. |

body. A spastic child has a rigid body, is **stiff** and has slow, difficult movements due to the stiffness in his muscles. Certain positions and situations may affect the level of spasticity. For instance, excitement or distress may trigger **abnormal reflexive responses** in the whole body and increase stiffness [7, 12, 15]. Degrees of spasticity may range from mild, moderate to severe based on limb involvement [7, 12, 15].

• *Spastic Hemiplegic*: One side of the body is spastic; usually the arm is more affected than the leg (Fig. 3.2).
• *Spastic Diplegia*: Both legs are affected. The term "scissoring" refers to the crossed leg position (Fig. 3.3). This is the result of stiffness of the muscles in the hips and the legs which make the legs turn inward at the level of the knees [7, 12, 15].
• *Spastic Quadriplegia*: All limbs are affected. Children become unable to walk properly (Fig. 3.4). Often, these children present with mental retardation, speech difficulty and seizure disorder.

*Athetoid or Dyskinetic Cerebral Palsy*

The Centers for Disease Control and Prevention estimate that around 10–20 % of children with cerebral palsy are athetoid or dyskinetic [15]. Athetoid or dyskinesis refers to an uncontrollable **alteration of**

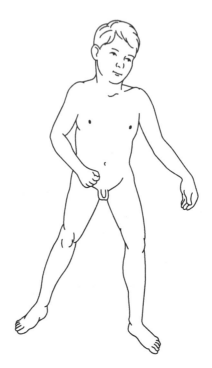

**Fig. 3.2** *Spastic Hemiplegia*

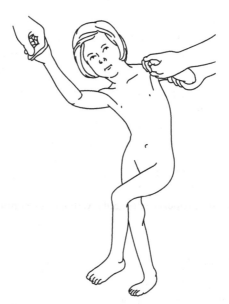

**Fig. 3.3** *Spastic Diplegia*

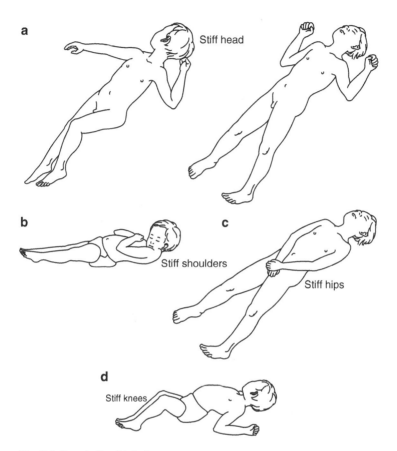

**Fig. 3.4** *Spastic Quadriplegia*

**muscle tension in the body from loose to stiff**. Children with athetoid or dyskinetic cerebral palsy often portray a variety of uncontrolled movements from sudden quick movements (Fig. 3.5), as a cause of stiffness, to slow fluid movements, as a cause of a softening in muscle tension [7, 12, 15]. Because of their variable muscle tone, children with athetoid CP have difficulty in walking and sitting. **Talking and swallowing** are also affected due to fluctuation in tone of facial muscles, making it difficult to communicate and eat alone.

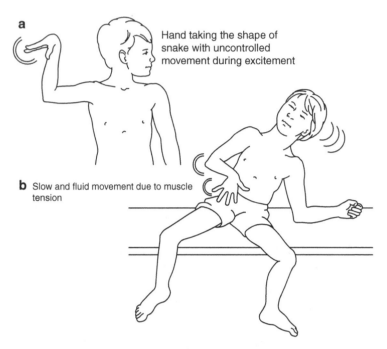

**Fig. 3.5** Athetoid or Dyskinetic Cerebral Palsy

*Ataxic Cerebral Palsy*

The Centers for Disease Control and Prevention estimate that around 5–10 % of children with cerebral palsy are ataxic [15]. Ataxic cerebral palsy is characterized by low muscle tone with **difficulty in balance and coordination** (Fig. 3.6) resulting in difficulty in sitting, standing and walking. Children with ataxic CP require more concentration and longer time to complete certain tasks such as writing [7, 15].

## *What to Do When Cerebral Palsy Is Suspected or Diagnosed?*

- Once CP is suspected it is important to act on it **as early as possible**
- **Working** on an abnormal motor function and posture **early on even before complete diagnosis** has been shown to improve functional outcome [6].
- It is important to **promote functional capacity** rather than to focus on fixing the underlying disease; i.e., the focus should be

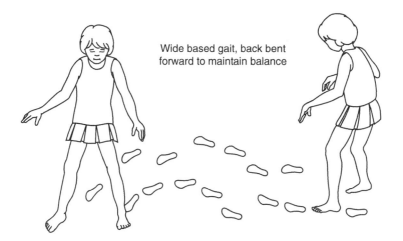

Wide based gait, back bent forward to maintain balance

**Fig. 3.6** Ataxia with difficulty in balance and coordination

on improving spasticity, hypertonicity, or abnormal reflex functions [2].

- Interventions geared towards manipulating the child's environment in order to give him or her better mobility has been shown to affect positively the child's language, exploration, physical, and social function [2].
- Physical therapy using the Bobath technique known also as neuro-developmental treatment (NDT) is currently considered to be controversial. NDT was initially presumed to inhibit abnormal muscle tone and facilitate normal movement. NDT was supposed to reduce tonic reflexes and spasm by using special exercises and positions that can ultimately, with repetitions, reduce abnormal functionality in patients with CP [28] Currently, there are concerns about its efficacy and even safety; wrong application of NDT in children can be dangerous and thus, can cause epiphysis injuries during child growth [29]. However, concerns about efficacy of physical therapy methods have been raised not only about this method but also about other methods due to the general lack of well-designed long term studies in this field [30].

Early Intervention for Cerebral Palsy

Children with cerebral palsy are **prone to be in abnormal positions** (Fig. 3.7) due to the increased or decreased muscle tone which may be encountered in spastic, athetoid, or ataxic cerebral

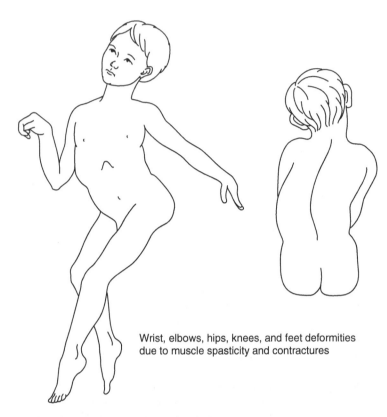

Wrist, elbows, hips, knees, and feet deformities
due to muscle spasticity and contractures

**Fig. 3.7** Abnormal positions of children with cerebral palsy

palsy. Early intervention has been shown to **prevent spasticity and improve functionality** [2–5] (Table 3.3). Interventions can range from occupation and physical therapy to medication and simple exercises that may be used on a **daily basis** by parents in order to supplement the medical treatment that their children may be receiving [12, 16, 17].

### *Interventions to Achieve Better Positions*

Simple and effective exercises and interventions to improve the functionality of children with cerebral palsy aim at **correcting the child's abnormal positions** by placing her in settings that will help maintain normal positions for a certain amount of time. It is important to aim for positions that keep the child's head, body, and limbs straight instead of bent or twisted. Table 3.4 shows examples of different

**Table 3.2** GMFCS of Children 2 to 4 years

| Level I | • Floor sit with both hands free to manipulate objects.<br>• Move in and out of floor sitting and standing without adult assistance.<br>• Walking is the preferred method of mobility without assistive mobility device. |
|---|---|
| Level II | • Floor sit but may have difficulty with balance when both hands are free to manipulate objects.<br>• Movements in and out of sitting performed without adult assistance.<br>• Pull to stand on a stable surface.<br>• Crawl on hands and knees with a reciprocal pattern, cruise holding onto furniture<br>• Walking using mobility device is the preferred methods of mobility. |
| Level III | • Maintain floor sitting by "W-sitting" and may require adult assistance to assume sitting position.<br>• Creep on stomach or crawl on hands and knees as primary methods of self-mobility.<br>• May pull to stand on a stable surface and cruise short distances.<br>• May walk short distances indoors using a hand-held mobility device (walker) with adult assistance for steering and turning. |
| Level IV | • Floor sit when placed, but unable to maintain alignment and balance without use of hands for support.<br>• Frequently require adaptive equipment for sitting and standing.<br>• Self-mobility for short distances achieved by rolling, creeping on stomach, or crawling on hands and knees without reciprocal leg movement. |
| Level V | • Physical impairments restrict voluntary control of movement and ability to maintain antigravity head and trunk postures.<br>• All areas of motor function are limited in sitting and standing.<br>• Functional limitations not fully compensated by adaptive equipment and assistive technology.<br>• No means of independent movement.<br>• Achieve self-mobility using powered wheelchair with extensive adaptations. |

positions that may be adapted while the child is going through daily activities such as lying, sitting, standing, playing, sleeping, and others.

### *General Guidelines About Body Position During Eating and Drinking*

1. The **stability of the head and trunk** is important for safety while eating.
2. The capability **to control mouth movement** during eating and drinking depends on **stability and alignment of the head** and

**Table 3.3** Types of CP and physical therapy

| Type of CP | Clinical characteristics | Goal of physical therapy |
|---|---|---|
| Spastic | • Increased muscle tone<br>• Increased deep tendon reflex<br>• Tightness and rigidity of the limbs<br>• *Diplegia: "Scissoring" of the legs*<br>• *Hemiplegia: affecting limbs on one side of the body*<br>• *Quadriplegia: affecting all four limbs* | • Prevent contraction of spastic muscles<br>• Strengthen weak muscles<br>Increase mobility |
| Hypotonic | • Diminished muscle tone<br>• Head lag<br>• Flaccidity and inability to control limb movements | • Strengthen muscles<br>• Improve posture<br>• Improve speech, swallowing, and breathing |
| Choreo-athetotic | • Uncontrollable writhing movements in arm/legs activated by emotions/ stress<br>• Variable muscle tones | • Prevent contraction of muscles |
| Ataxic | • Uncoordinated movements<br>• Tremor<br>• Loss of power | • Improve balance<br>• Develop reflexes<br>• Prevent atrophy in unused muscles |
| Dystonic | • Strained muscle contractions<br>• Twisting and repetitive movements<br>• Abnormal postures (some cases) | • Improve posture<br>• Prevent contraction of muscles |
| Ballismic | • Uncoordinated jerky movements of the limbs | • Prevent contraction of muscles |
| Mixed | • Multiple symptoms of the above mentioned types of CP | • All of the above |

**Table 3.4** Positioning during daily activities

| Position | Aim | Technique | Example | Indication | Figures |
|---|---|---|---|---|---|
| Lying/ Sleeping | Break spasticity | – Bend a child forward over an object while lying<br>– Help child lie down in a bent position | – Bend child over a large ball<br>– Place child in a tire swing<br>– Place in a hammock | – Spastic cerebral palsy<br>– Athetoid cerebral palsy | Fig. 3.8 |
| | Prevent "scissoring" | Keep child in a position where his/her legs are held apart | – Hold apart child's legs by thick diapers or thick layers of clothing<br>– Pin child's legs apart | – Spastic cerebral palsy (diplegia, quadriplegia)<br>– Other cases in which "scissoring" is apparent | Fig. 3.9 |
| | Strengthen muscles to lift head | Position child to help him use arms to lift head up | Place pillow or soft object under child's stomach to higher him off the ground and facilitate the lifting of his head | – Athetoid cerebral palsy<br>– Ataxic cerebral palsy<br>– Other cases of children with low muscle tone | Fig. 3.10 |
| | Straighten head position | Position child to lie with head opposite to the side which it is usually turned to | Position pillows behind child's neck | – Spastic cerebral palsy (quadriplegia)<br>– Athetoid cerebral palsy | Fig. 3.11 |
| | Straighten body | Position child that arches backward on his side in a lying position | Position pillows around the child | Spastic cerebral palsy (quadriplegia) | Fig. 3.12 |

(continued)

**Table 3.4** (continued)

| Position | Aim | Technique | Example | Indication | Figures |
|---|---|---|---|---|---|
| Sitting | Correct for abnormal body positions | Seat child in position countering the abnormal position he is usually in | – Child with legs pressed together and arms turned in should be seated with legs apart and arms turned outward<br>– Child with legs apart and shoulders pushed back should be seated legs together and body bent forward | – Spastic cerebral palsy (diplegia, quadriplegia)<br>– Athetoid cerebral palsy | Fig. 3.13 |
| | Correct sitting positions for children with balance problems | Balance problems cause children to sit with their legs in the form of a "W"—position child to sit with legs spread out forward<br>*N.B. If child cannot use hands while sitting except in W position, then it should be allowed* | – Place toys in between the child's legs to keep the knees apart<br>– Sit child on a toy horse to keep legs straight and apart | – Spastic cerebral palsy (diplegia, quadriplegia)<br>– Athetoid cerebral palsy<br>– Ataxic cerebral palsy<br>– Other cases of children with balance problems | Fig. 3.14 |
| | Improve seating of children with low muscle tone | Help child remain seated in an upright position | – Seat child and help keep his position using barriers on both sides<br>– Seat child in a car seat while playing | – Athetoid cerebral palsy<br>– Ataxic cerebral palsy<br>– Other cases of children with low muscle tones | Fig. 3.15 |

| Standing | Improve child's balance in standing positions | Assisting child with his balance decreases the tightening and tensing of muscles and helps him stand straight | – Give child a stick to hold onto with both hands while standing and maintain balance from other side of the stick | – Spastic cerebral palsy (hemiplegia, diplegia) | Fig. 3.16 |
| | | | – Give child two sticks to hold on either side while walking | – Athetoid cerebral palsy | |
| | | | | – Ataxic cerebral palsy | |
| | Prevent body deformities and encourage growth and strengthening of legs | Place child who cannot stand alone in a standing frame for a couple of hours | Logs or a play horse can also be used instead of a standing frame | – Spastic cerebral palsy (quadriplegia) | Fig. 3.17 |
| | | | | – Severe athetoid cerebral palsy | |
| Rolling/ twisting | Loosen body muscles | Encourage child to roll and twist with help and with toys | – Help roll and twist child's body | – Spastic cerebral palsy (diplegia, quadriplegia) | Fig. 3.18 |
| | | | – Place toys out of reach for child to twist and reach out for | – Athetoid cerebral palsy | |

(continued)

**Table 3.4** (continued)

| Position | Aim | Technique | Example | Indication | Figures |
|---|---|---|---|---|---|
| Carrying | Correct for abnormal positions during carrying | Carry the child in positions that oppose the abnormal positions he is usually in | – Child with straightened legs and bent arms should be carried with bent legs and straightened arms | – Spastic cerebral palsy (diplegia, quadriplegia) – Athetoid cerebral palsy | Fig. 3.19 |
| | | | – Child that is usually curled up should be carried in a position that straightens his body out | – Ataxic cerebral palsy | Fig. 3.20 |
| | | | – Child that usually arches backward and straightens out should be carried with legs spread out and shoulders pushed back | | Fig. 3.20 |
| Hand exercises | Improve function of hands and fingers | Encourage the use of hands and fingers when playing in following areas:<br>• Grasping<br>• Releasing<br>• Squeezing | – Give child paper to crumple up, throw and pick up again – Give child a book or magazine to turn pages – Encourage child to participate in getting dressed | Spastic cerebral palsy (hemiplegia) Athetoid cerebral palsy | Fig. 3.21 |
| Moving about | Correct abnormal positions for children who cannot walk | Correct abnormal position of children who cannot move but can move around using help through positioning on different aids | Play horse Toy car Wheelboards Wheelchairs | – Spastic cerebral palsy (hemiplegia, diplegia, quadriplegia) – Athetoid cerebral palsy – Ataxic cerebral palsy | Fig. 3.22 |

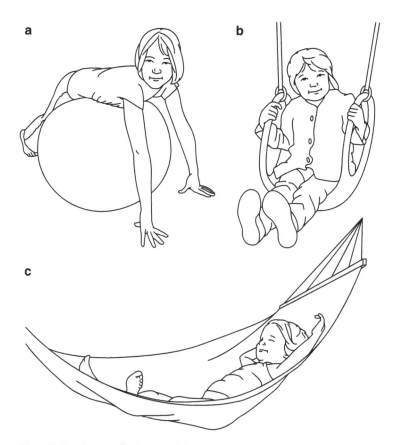

**Fig. 3.8** Positions to alleviate spasticity: (**a**) lying over a large ball, (**b**) using tire as a swing, (**c**) using a hammock

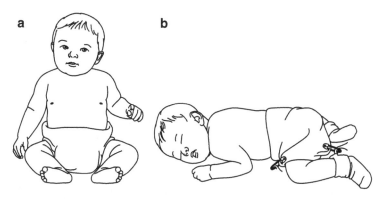

**Fig. 3.9** Positions to prevent "scissoring". (**a**) use thick or double diapers to keep legs apart, (**b**) use pins to keep legs apart

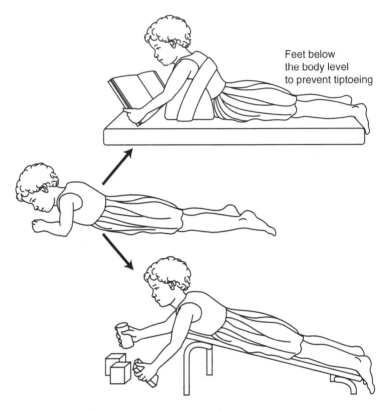

Feet below
the body level
to prevent tiptoeing

**Fig. 3.10** Muscle strengthening positions

trunk's position. There should be **symmetry of the body** on both sides with the head maintained in the middle.

3. The **neck** should be put **backwards in a flat** way in all positions of eating whether in sitting, standing, or semilying.

4. The child should feel **relaxed and comfortable** during eating and drinking. The feeling of tension and worrisome increases muscular tension and the appearance of involuntary movements which make the eating and drinking process difficult.

5. The **person helping** in the feeding process is better **seated facing the child, helping the child maintain the head** in its best position. This allows **continuous eye contact** with the child thus

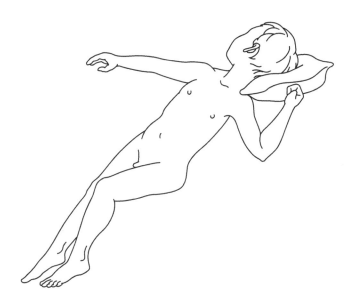

**Fig. 3.11** Pillow support to straighten head

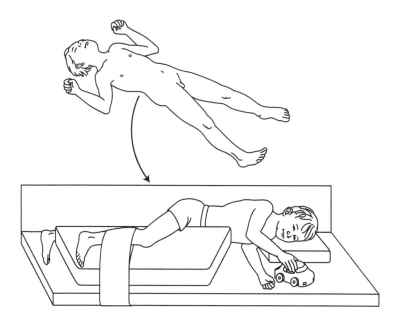

**Fig. 3.12** Different matt positions for body support

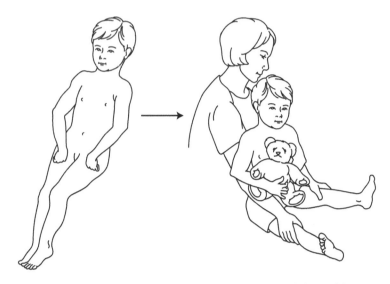

**Fig. 3.13** Avoid abnormal body position and support correct sitting positions

receiving his needs and desires; in addition the child would be able to see the food coming to him.

The child's feet should **be fixed on the floor** in order to feel safe (Table 3.5).

## *Therapy for Spasticity and Dystonia in CP Patients*

Several treatment options are available for spasticity and dystonia in cerebral palsy, ranging from oral medications to local intramuscular injections to surgical interventions [18–24].

**Oral medications** include baclofen, diazepam, dantrolene sodium, and alpha-2 noradrenergic agonist (Tizanidine) for spasticity and dopeminergic and anticholinergic medications for dystonia [18, 22]. Although oral medications are the least invasive, they often have **undesirable side effects** [20].

Injection therapies include **Botulinum toxin** (BoNT) which promotes muscle denervation via axonal degeneration resulting in

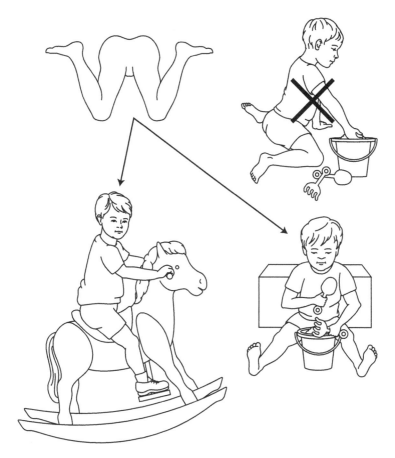

**Fig. 3.14** Tips to use for correct sitting positions

transient muscle paralysis leading to a **balance in the muscle forces thus improving motor function**; in addition, this leads to **decreased spasticity** and muscle pain [18, 21, 25]. BoNT injections decrease hypertonicity from a period of few weeks to 2 years without inducing any major side effects and is **generally well tolerated** when given in appropriate doses [18, 25].

**Intrathecal Baclofen Infusion** (ITB) involves the **implantation of a pump** providing direct infusion of baclofen intrathecally. Baclofen acts as a **muscle relaxant** and antispastic agent that improves the range of motion and facilitates movements of spastic

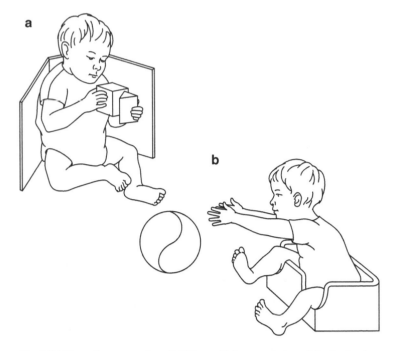

**Fig. 3.15** Tips to improve seating of children with low muscle tone: (**a**) using barriers on both sides, (**b**) using car seat while playing

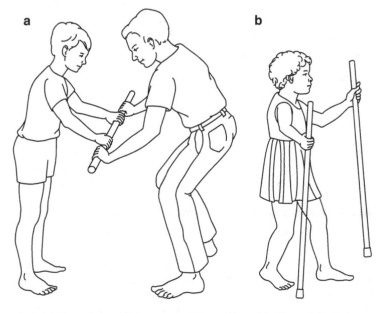

**Fig. 3.16** Tips to improve balance in standing positions: (**a**) using a stick to balance, (**b**) using two sticks to walk

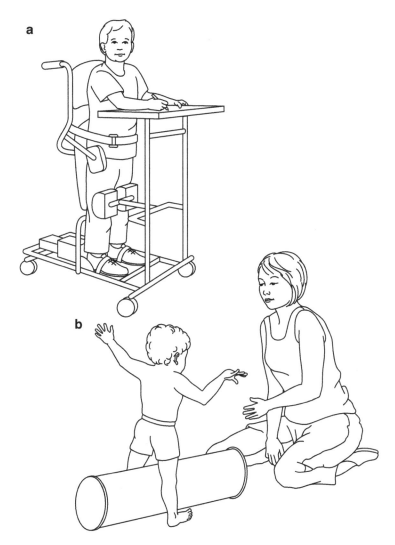

**Fig. 3.17** Methods to encourage growth and strength: (**a**) using standing frame, (**b**) using logs or play horse

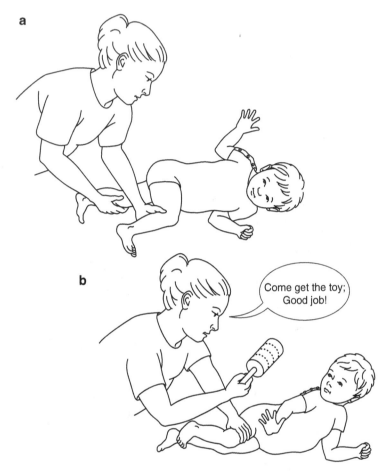

**Fig. 3.18** Methods to help loosening body muscles: (**a**) Rolling and twisting child's body, (**b**) Placing a toy out of reach and stimulating child to reach

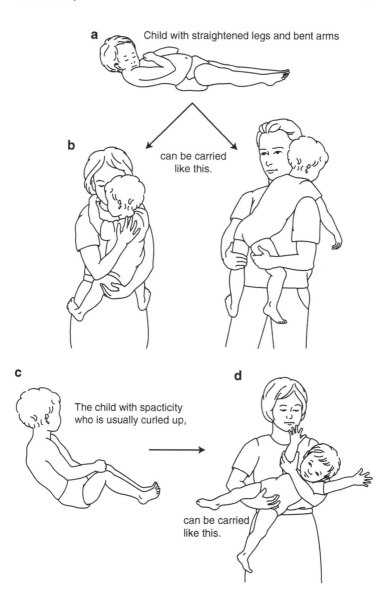

**a** Child with straightened legs and bent arms

**b** can be carried like this.

**c** The child with spacticity who is usually curled up,

**d** can be carried like this.

**Fig. 3.19** Correct embracement for abnormal positions

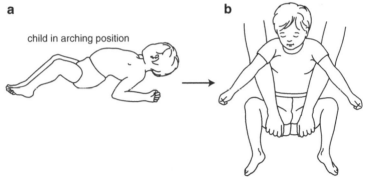

**a** child in arching position

**b** Child can be carried with legs spread out and shoulders pushed back

**Fig. 3.20** Tips to correct abnormal position

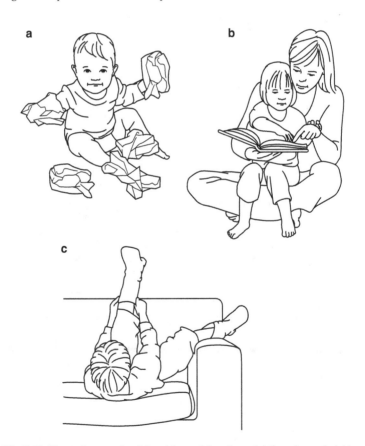

**Fig. 3.21** Tips to improve hands' and fingers' functions: (**a**) throwing and picking up papers, (**b**) turning book pages, (**c**) getting dressed by himself

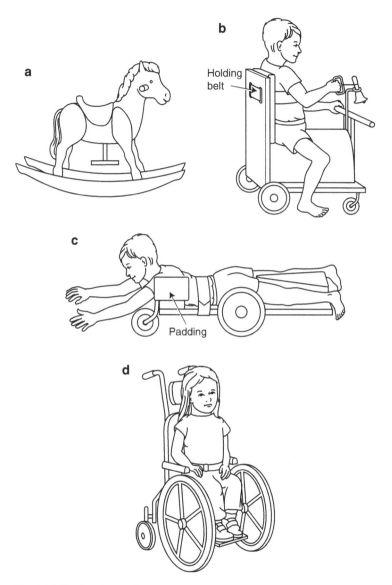

**Fig. 3.22** Tips for abnormal positions: (**a**) using play horse, (**b**) using a toy car, (**c**) using wheel boards, (**d**) using wheelchair

**Table 3.5** Useful tools to be used at home

| Tools | Description | Picture |
|---|---|---|
| Padded tools | | |
| Floor mats | • Hard padded mats are best<br>• Easily cleaned after usage<br>• Child feels safe while moving | Fig. 3.23 |
| Padded tables | • Low tables, not exceeding 45 cm<br>• Useful for older children's activities | Fig. 3.24 |
| Helpful tools during lying | | |
| Cylindrical rolls or ball | • Sponge with plastic cover<br>• Used for lifting body parts<br>• Easy to move<br>• Use appropriate size for each child | Fig. 3.25 |
| Sliding wedges | • Used to support the child's body<br>• Non movable<br>• Useful for positioning at home | Fig. 3.26 |
| Pilow/sliding wedge | • Beneficial for a short period<br>• Used for children capable of head lifting<br>• Sand bags could be used for side support | Fig. 3.27 |
| Side-lying board | • Important for hypotonic children<br>• Beneficial for spastic children with arching or those who do not tolerate lying on their stomachs | Fig. 3.28 |
| Sitting and standing | | |
| Benches and stools | • Wooden tools to help child move from sitting to standing and vice versa | Fig. 3.29 |
| Standing tables | • Tables with variable heights<br>• Can be controlled electrically | Fig. 3.30 |

| | | |
|---|---|---|
| Special chairs | • Adjustable to child's needs<br>• Should be comfortable and allow child to be active | Fig. 3.31 |
| Reclining chair | • Supports the child in the reclining position.<br>• Neck pillow needed for head support<br>• Feet board needed for feet support<br>• Belts between the thighs may be needed to keep pelvis in backward position | Fig. 3.32 |
| Upright chair and table | • Used for children who can partially control their head and trunk<br>• A table at the level of the chest can be added as well as knee blocks to push the pelvis backwards | Fig. 3.33 |
| Prone angle chair (forward tilting) | • Used for children who feel more comfortable sitting with forward tilting<br>• Front support at chest level is needed | Fig. 3.34 |
| Standing frames | • Upright standing boards.<br>• Prone angle standing boards with forward tilting | Fig. 3.35<br>Fig. 3.36 |
| Inserts | • Used for better sitting positions into wheelchairs or pushchairs<br>• Allows a better control of body positions | Fig. 3.37 |
| Walking | | |
| Walking aids | • Useful to help child carry body weight by hands and arms to facilitate movement | Fig. 3.38 |
| Splints for legs and arms | • Useful for straightening extremities<br>• Used for a short period of time | Fig. 3.39 |
| Ride-on walkers | • Three wheel bicycle<br>• Wooden horse or walker with wheels | Fig. 3.40 |
| Bathroom | | |
| Toilet chairs | • Support materials placed on top of toilet seats<br>• Provide support during toilet training and subsequent use | Fig. 3.41 |
| Bathing tools | • Secure base to support child in sitting position during bath | Fig. 3.42 |

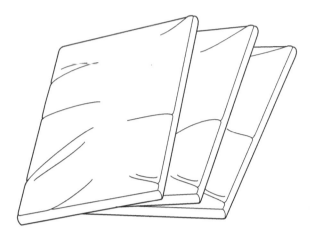

**Fig. 3.23** Floor mats

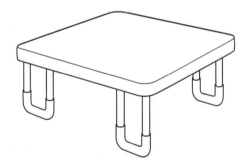

**Fig. 3.24** Padded table

children [18–20, 23]. Its use reduces the need for orthopedic surgery [18–20]. ITB has **fewer side effects** than oral medications because of the lower dose used; however, potential complications associated with implantation and high cost are a drawback [23]. In parallel to ITB before and after infusion, **physical therapy still plays a major role in management** [23].

**Surgical therapies** include:

• **Rhizotomy** and other orthopedic corrective surgeries for spastic CP [18].

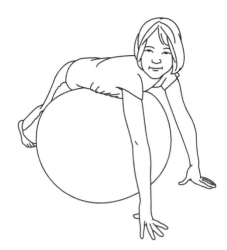

**Fig. 3.25** Rolling ball

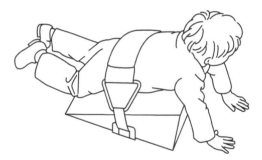

**Fig. 3.26** Sliding wedge

- **Ablative thalamic surgery** for cerebral palsy with dystonia [19, 22].
- Other therapies include **deep brain stimulation**, using high-frequency electrical stimulation of the cerebral structures which has been shown to be effective in cerebral palsy with dystonia [22, 24].

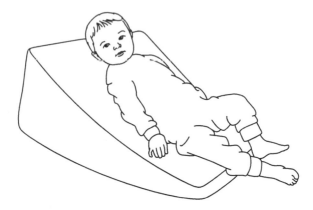

**Fig. 3.27** Pillow or sliding wedge

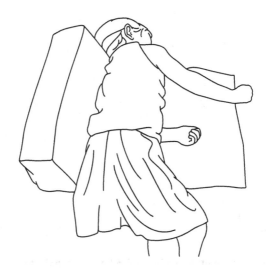

**Fig. 3.28** Side-lying board

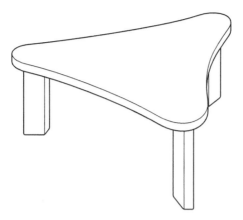

**Fig. 3.29** Low sitting table

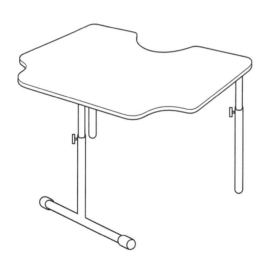

**Fig. 3.30** Standing / sitting table with special anchor

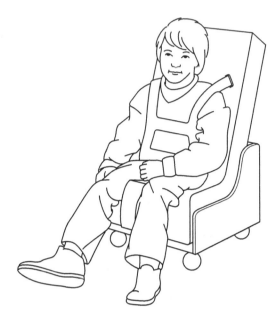

**Fig. 3.31** Special chair

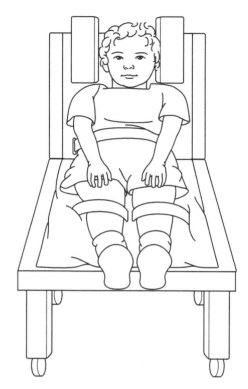

**Fig. 3.32** Reclining chair

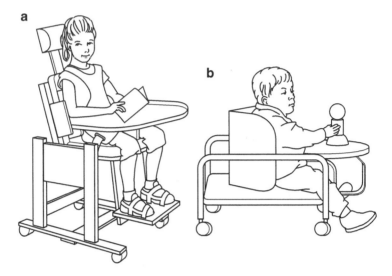

**Fig. 3.33** Upright chairs and tables: (**a**) child sitting in a chair with head and trunk support, (**b**) child using a table on wheels with back support

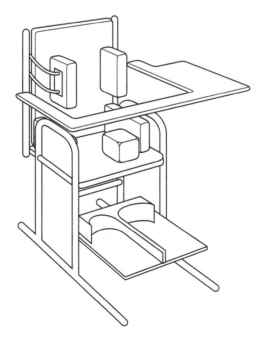

**Fig. 3.34** Prone angle chair with forward tilting

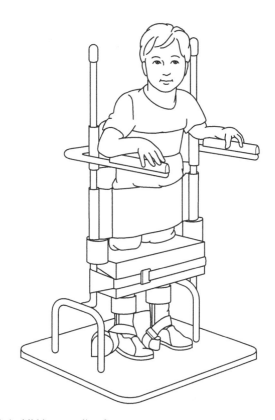

**Fig. 3.35** A child in a standing frame

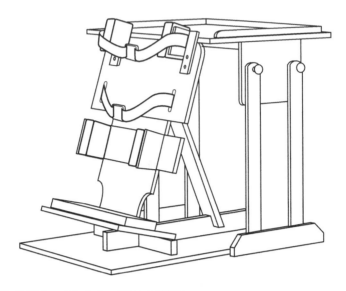

**Fig. 3.36** Insert for better sitting positions

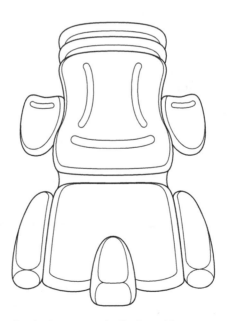

**Fig. 3.37** Insert allowing better control of body positions

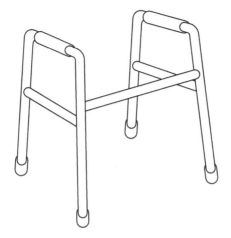

**Fig. 3.38** Walking aid

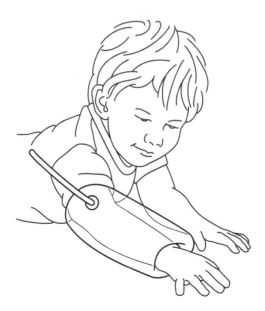

**Fig. 3.39** Splint for the arm

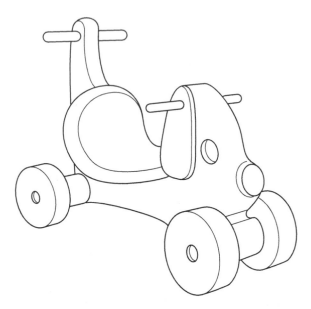

**Fig. 3.40** Ride-on walker

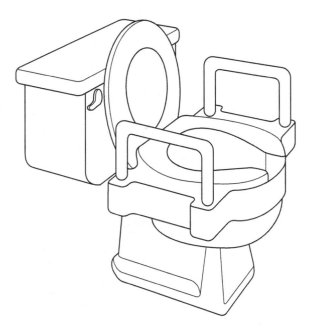

**Fig. 3.41** Bathroom Support materials to be placed on toilet seat top

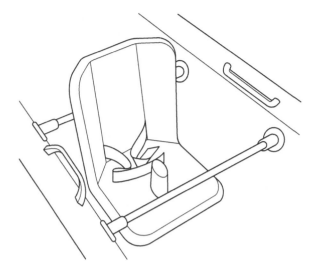

**Fig. 3.42** Bathing tool with a secure base

# Other Disorders Affecting Motor Development

## *Down Syndrome*

Down syndrome or trisomy 21 is the most common chromosomal abnormality. It is characterized by distinct facial features, delays in early child development, and mental retardation [25–27].

- Typical physical features are flat face, slanting eyes with epicanthal folds, large tongue, small ears and mouth, stubby fingers, broad hands, feet and neck, decreased muscle tone, and short stature.
- Associated anomalies may include congenital heart defects, specifically AV canal; duodenal atresia; and hypothyroidism.
- Early development is particularly delayed in gross motor function, as well as cognitive language and social delay [6, 25–27].

Early intervention focusing on enhancing motor skills and language development has been deemed effective in many studies [1, 6, 25, 31]. For example, early interventions help prevent complications resulting from abnormal positions related to decreased muscle tone [6]. Activities that can be done at home may include [6, 31]:

- Engagement in physical activity by using games that require movement
- Active interaction with parents, for example, using board games for older children, creating new games, avoid directive and nonresponsive interaction
- Use of manual signs for preverbal communication
- Encourage talking/verbalization by asking the child for a response
- Engage in social activity, playing with other children
- Enroll in KG/school as early as possible

## *Duchenne Muscular Dystrophy*

Duchenne Muscular Dystrophy (DMD) is a progressive disease caused by a sex-linked recessive gene resulting in the absence of the protein dystrophin from the body. The disease mainly affects males and is characterized by gradual muscle degeneration. Muscle cells in the body are gradually replaced by fat cells and fibrous tissue leading to difficulties in movements of arms and legs and general weakness in the body. As the disease progresses it affects the heart and diaphragm, causing heart and respiratory failure [26, 32, 33].

Early symptoms of DMD can be detected as early as 3 years of age, when the child begins losing motor skills, often manifested as [27, 32]:

- New onset of clumsiness, awkwardness, or frequent falls
- Tiptoe walking
- Difficulty in climbing stairs
- Quickly getting tired

Later as disease progresses, calf muscle enlargement is observed, along with:

- "Gower's Maneuver"—child uses all fours to get off the floor pushes on thighs to straighten into standing position
- Standing posture—child tends to sway back with protrusion of abdomen

Early intervention for children with DMD may not prevent further muscle loss, however it improves muscle strength and function and helps prevent secondary complications including decreased respiratory function, scoliosis, and contractures [27, 32, 33].

Management of DMD involves treatment with glucocorticosteroids, physiotherapy, and the use of equipment as needed [32, 33]:

- Glucocorticosteroid treatment usually given as low-doses under supervision of a neurologist upon disease confirmation [32, 33].
- Physiotherapy: stretching exercises are effective in enhancing and maintaining muscle function, delaying contractures and preventing scoliosis [27, 32].
- Equipments: provision of equipments such as ankle–foot–orthoses (AFO) help delaying contractures, and knee–ankle–foot–orthoses (KAFO) that are effective in prolonging the walking and standing ability. In addition, proper seating equipment helps in providing necessary postural support in order to prevent scoliosis [27, 32].

## Guillain–Barré Syndrome

Guillain–Barré syndrome (GBS), also known as acute inflammatory demyelinating polyneuropathy (AIDP), is an autoimmune disorder characterized by "demyelination" of nerves and causing muscle weakness [34, 35]. The disease may occur at any age, however in children close to one-third of the cases occur before the age of 3 years [35]. Symptoms are rapidly progressive, at times becoming severe in matter of days to a couple of weeks and include [34–36]:

- Pain (especially in the back and lower limbs)—very important symptom that is usually under-identified for children
- Symmetric muscle weakness (both sides of the body) or loss of function (paralysis)
- Areflexia (loss of neurologic and muscle stretch reflexes)
- Ascending paralysis (loss of muscle function beginning at the lower extremities and spreading to upper extremities)
- Ataxia (loss of movement coordination)

Upon diagnosis, children are hospitalized for pain management and other therapeutic and supportive treatments such as antiinflammatory medications [34–36], plasmapherisis, and

Intravenous Immunoglobulin (IVIG) therapies which have been found to be effective in reducing the severity and duration of GBS symptoms [37, 38, 34, 35].

After treatment, the following may be initiated in order to prevent complications [34–36]:

- Physical and occupational therapy—exercise muscles and joints to maintain mobility, ensure proper body positioning and breathing support and manage pain
- Nutrition management—maintaining appropriate caloric intake in order to avoid accelerated muscle catabolism (degeneration)
- Continuous schooling—adopting "home" schooling, especially when children are hospitalized for long periods of time, continuing their education is considered an important intervention

## *Poliomyelitis (Polio)*

Poliomyelitis, or Polio, is a condition occurring after infection with poliovirus, causing acute flaccid paralysis [39, 40]. Poliovirus is transmitted through the fecal–oral route and is known to affect mostly young children, pregnant women, and elderly people [39, 40]. Polio is preventable through proper immunization [39]. Oral Polio Vaccine (OPV) has been replaced by Inactivated Polio Vaccine (IPV) in developed countries where most cases of polio occur following vaccination with OPV. Wild polio is still present in developing countries and therefore vaccination in those countries is mainly through OPV [41].

Symptoms include [39, 40]:

- Fever
- Malaise
- Headache
- Vomiting
- Limb, back, and neck pain
- Muscle stiffness, pain and/or weakness, in some cases leading to permanent paralysis

Interventions for children affected with polio include analgesics and/or heat therapy in order to decrease limb pain and muscle stiffness and physical therapy in order to enhance muscle strength and function [40].

## *Stroke*

Strokes occur when a sudden occlusion or rupture occurs in the cerebral arteries or veins causing damage to the Central Nervous System (CNS). Strokes in children and infants are rare; the diagnosis is often delayed or under-recognized. Children suffering from strokes have different risk factors compared to adults, and their clinical symptoms and outcomes are also distinct [42].

Risk factors associated with strokes in infants and children include:

- Cardiac disease, congenital or acquired
- Metabolic, hematological, or coagulation disorders (dislipidemias, mitochondrial encephalopathy, sickle cell disease, leukemia, Antithrombin III deficiency, Protein S and C deficiency, etc.)
- Postinfectious vasculitis (meningitis, varicella, mycoplasma, HIV)
- Adverse drug reaction
- Maternal factors (vasospasm due to migraine or drug use, autoimmunity)

Clinical signs and symptoms of stroke in children are not specific and often overlap with those of other neurological and non-CNS-related disorders. Children should be screened for strokes when presenting with any of the following [42]:

- Sudden onset of weakness, speech, or visual disturbances
- Seizures in the neonatal period or postcardiac surgery
- Decrease in level of consciousness with presence of headache
- Neurological deficits

Treatment recommendations are based on adult treatment standards since no standards are available for children. The basis of the management lies in treating the underlying condition. Aspirin is widely used as an anticoagulant [42].

Nearly 50–85 % of children diagnosed with a stroke have long-term disabilities such as seizures, difficulties in motor, and behavioral and learning abilities [42].

Early intervention can help stroke victims regain movement, speech, and thinking; with occupational and physical therapy, the physical, mental, and cognitive challenges are addressed; therefore, rehabilitation is recommended soon after stroke occurs. In addition, rehabilitation helps prevent future strokes and avoid complications.

According to the American Occupational Therapy Association, occupational therapy started at an early stage of recovery is associated with more rapid recovery [43]. The intervention is focused on helping the child regain independence in performing daily activities and regaining previously learnt skills. A holistic approach is preferred in which the patient's needs, limitations, requests, activities, and environment are taken into account. Physical therapists focus on impaired limbs, teaching alternate ways of accomplishing tasks with new deficits and providing ongoing exercise programs [43]. Home equipments that can assist the person in caring for themselves may be recommended by the occupational therapist.

# References

1. Staudt M. Brain plasticity following early life brain injury. Semin Perinatol. 2010;34:87–92.
2. Rosenbaum P. Cerebral palsy: what parents and doctors want to know? Br Med J. 2003;326:970–4.
3. Russman BS, Ashwal S. Evaluation of the child with cerebral palsy. Semin Pediatr Neurol. 2004;11(1):47–57.
4. Palisano RJ, Snider LM, Orlin MN. Recent advances in physical and occupational therapy for children with cerebral palsy. Semin Pediatr Neurol. 2004;11(1):66–77.
5. Damiano DL. Activity, activity, activity: rethinking our physical therapy approach to cerebral palsy. Phys Ther. 2006;86(11):1534–40.
6. Mahoney G, Robinson C, Fewell RR. The effects of early motor intervention on children with down syndrome or cerebral palsy: a field-based study. J Dev Behav Pediatr. 2001;22(3):153–62.
7. Werner D. Disabled village children – a guide for community health workers, rehabilitation workers, and families. 2nd ed. Palo Alto, CA: The Hesperian Foundation; 2009.
8. Rosenbaum P. The definition and classification of cerebral palsy: are we any further ahead in 2006? NeoReviews. 2006;7:e569–74.
9. Shevell MI, Bodensteiner JB. Cerebral palsy: defining the problem. Semin Pediatr Neurol. 2004;11(1):2–4.
10. Shevell MI. The "bermuda triangle" of neonatal neurology: cerebral palsy, neonatal encephalopathy, and intrapartum asphyxia. Semin Pediatr Neurol. 2004;11(1):24–30.
11. Centers for Disease Control and Prevention (CDC) (2006) Learn the signs, act early: cerebral palsy fact sheet. http://www.cdc.gov/actearly. Accessed 17 Nov 2010.
12. Tilton AH. Management of spasticity in children with cerebral palsy. Semin Pediatr Neurol. 2004;11(1):58–65.

13. Palisano R, Rosenbaum P, Bartlett D. and Livingston M (2007) Gross motor function classification system – expanded and revised. Can child centre for childhood disability research, McMaster University. http://motorgrowth.canchild.ca/en/GMFCS/resources/GMFCS-ER.pdf. Accessed 13 Dec 2010.

14. Palisano R, Rosenbaum P, Walter S, Russell D, Wood E, Galuppi B. Development and reliability of a system to classify gross motor function in children with cerebral palsy. Dev Med Child Neurol. 1997;39:214–23.

15. Centers for Disease Control and Prevention (CDC) (2004) Cerebral palsy. http://www.cdc.gov/ncbddd/dd/cp2.htm. Accessed 17 Nov 2010.

16. Krigger KW. Cerebral palsy: an overview. Am Fam Physician. 2006;73(1):91–100.

17. Taylor F, National Institute of Neurological Disorders and Stroke (U.S.), Office of Science and Health Reports. Cerebral palsy: hope through research. Bethesda, MD: The Institute; 2001. Accessed http://www.ninds.nih.gov/disorders/cerebral_palsy/detail_cerebral_palsy.htm#154403104.

18. Verrotti A, Greco R, Spalice A, Chiarelli F, Iannetti P. Pharmacotherapy of spasticity in children with cerebral palsy. Pediatr Neurol. 2006;34(1):1–6.

19. Gerszten PC, Albright L, Johnstone GF. Intrathecal baclofen infusion and subsequent orthopedic surgery in patients with spastic cerebral palsy. J Neurosurg. 1998;88(6):1009–13.

20. Nuttin B, Ivanhoe C, Albright L, Dimitrijevic M, Saltuari L. Intrathecal baclofen therapy for spasticity of cerebral origin: cerebral palsy and brain injury. Neuromodulation. 1999;2(2):120–32.

21. Koman LA, Smith BP, Balkrishnan R. Spasticity associated with cerebral palsy in children. Pediatric Drugs. 2003;5(1):11–23.

22. Bhidayasiri R. Dystonia: genetics and treatment update. Neurologist. 2006;12(2):74–85.

23. Barry MJ, Albright L, Shultz BL. Intrathecal baclofen therapy and the role of the physical therapist. Pediatr Phys Ther. 2000;12:77–86.

24. Roubertie A, Echenne B, Cif L, Vayssiere N, Hemm S, Coubes P. Treatment of early-onset dystonia: update and a new perspective. Childs Nerv Syst. 2000;16:334–40.

25. McLean WE, Hartley SL. Down syndrome. In: Salkind NJ, editor. Encyclopedia of human development (Vol I). Thousand Oaks, CA: Sage Publications; 2006. p. 394–6.

26. Hooper SR, Mills C. Developmental processes and factors affecting development. In: Hooper SR, Unmansky W, editors. Young children with special needs. New Jersey: Pearson Education; 2004. p. 38–89.

27. Dennis CW, Schlough KA. Gross motor development. In: Hooper SR, Unmansky W, editors. Young children with special needs. New Jersey: Pearson Education; 2004. p. 224–67.

28. Barry, M. (2001). Evidence-based practice in pediatric physical therapy. (11 ed., Vol. 9, p. 38). Ohio: Magazine of Physical Therapy..

29. Damiano, D., Dodd, K., & Taylor, N. (2002). Should we be testing and training muscle strength in cerebral palsy?. (44 ed., Vol. 1, pp. 68-72).

30. Mayston M. Evidence-based physical therapy for the management of children with cerebral palsy. Dev Med Child Neurol. 2005 Dec;47(12):795. PubMed PMID: 16288666.

31. Guralnick MJ. Early intervention for children with intellectual disabilities: current knowledge and future prospects. J Appl Res Intellect Disabil. 2005;18:313–24.

32. Bushby K, Bourke J, Bullock R, Eagle M, Gibson M, Quinby J. The multi-disciplinary management of Duchenne muscular dystrophy. Curr Paediatr. 2005;15(4):292–300.

33. Merlini L, Cicognani A, Malaspina E, Gennari M, Gnudi S, Talim B, Franzoni E. Early prednisone treatment in Duchenne muscular dystrophy. Muscle Nerve. 2003;27(2):222–7.

34. National Center for Biotechnology Information, U.S. National Library of Medicine (2010). Guillain–Barré syndrome. http://www.ncbi.nlm.nih.gov/pubmedhealth/PMH0001704/. Accessed 27 Apr 2011.

35. Ryan MM. Guillain–Barré syndrome in childhood. J Paediatr Child Health. 2005;41(5–6):237–41.

36. Sladky JT. Guillain–Barré syndrome in children. J Child Neurol. 2004;19(3):191–200.

37. Kanra G, Ozon A, Vajsar J, Castagna L, Secmeer G, Topaloglu H. Intravenous immunoglobulin treatment in children with Guillain–Barré syndrome. Eur J Paediatr Neurol. 1997;1:7–12.

38. Hughes RA, Swan AV, van Doorn PA. Intravenous immunoglobulin for Guillain–Barré syndrome. Cochrane Database Syst Rev 2010;(6):CD002063.

39. World Health Organization (2011) Poliomyelitis. http://www.who.int./topics/poliomyelitis/en/. Accessed 29 Apr 2011.

40. National Center for Biotechnology Information, U.S. National Library of Medicine (2009). Poliomyelitis. http://www.ncbi.nlm.nih.gov/pubmedhealth/PMH0002375/. Accessed 29 Apr 2011.

41. Center for Disease Control and Prevention (CDC) (2000). Polio vaccine: what you need to know. http://www.immunize.org/vis/ipv-00.pdf. Accessed 29 Apr 2011.

42. Mackay MT. Stroke in children. Aust Fam Physician. 2007;36(11):896–902.

43. Scheer J. Stroke recovery and OT: finding and using the evidence to inform practice. OT Practice. 2007;12(5):23–5.

# Chapter 4
# Enhancing Childhood Development in Children with Behavioral and Psychological Disorders

**Keywords** Behavioral disorder • Psychological disorder • Speech delay • Stuttering • Aggression • Behavioral management • Temper tantrums

Behavioral and psychological disorders in children may be difficult to recognize in the early years especially for first time parents. Normal variant of a specific behavior may be difficult to distinguish from a real behavioral problem. Furthermore, parents may feel uneasy or uncomfortable seeking professional help for the very young child. Therefore screening for these disorders should be an integral part of every well child check up since early identification, and referral for early intervention has been shown to impact significantly on the long-term outcome especially for children with Attention Deficit Hyperactivity Disorder (ADHD) for example [1]. In this chapter we highlight common behavioral and psychological problems that parents and primary healthcare provider may encounter in children at an early age. We also discuss various strategies to help

D. Sinno et al., *Enhancing Early Child Development:*
*A Handbook for Clinicians*, DOI 10.1007/978-1-4614-4827-3_4,
© Springer Science+Business Media, LLC 2013

parents manage these problems at home to minimize their negative impact on early child development.

> ### *Advise*
>
> *Provide the child with special attention through play and communication.*

> ### *Advise*
>
> *Children make mistakes while discovering things around them. Praise your child for good efforts*

## Speech Disorders

Language development and speech constitute major milestones in the normal development of a child. The four main areas of language development include semantics, morphology, syntax, and pragmatics [2, 3]. Language is communicated nonverbally through gestures and facial expressions and verbally through speech [3]. Communication skills begin to develop at birth through facial expressions, gestures, and primitive sounds with vocal development initiating during the first few months [4]. Below is a brief list of the milestones in speech development [2–5]:

- Birth–1 month: voice recognition, primitive sounds (cooing)
- 2–4 months: vowel-like sounds
- 5 months: single consonant and vowel sounds
- 6–9 months: babbling and jargon
- 10 months: production of sequential consonant and vowel sounds, echolalia
- 12–15 months: speak at least one word (3–4 clear words)
- 18–24 months: use a vocabulary of around 50 words
- 2–3 years: use a vocabulary of around 200 words

## *Delayed Speech*

Delay in speech may be attributed to several causes including environment and genetic or congenital factors [3, 5]. While a margin of delay in speech is usually normal if resolved by the age of 30 months, sometimes this delay is indicative of other underlying conditions [3]. Physical conditions attributed to speech delay may include hearing loss due to accumulation of fluids in the ears and sinuses or developmental disorders such as autism [5]. Recommended screenings for speech and language development are to take place at 9, 18, 24, and 30 months [4]. If screenings for associated disorders are not indicative, then environmental factors such as parental communication, house environment, witness of traumatic events, and others should be explored [3].

A stimulating environment for speech and language development at the house and during preschool is highly recommended for children with apparent speech delay, under the supervision of a speech therapist. Children should be talked to and encouraged to speak at all times [3, 5].

## *Stuttering*

Stuttering usually appears after the general phases of normal speech development at the ages of 2–4 years and affects boys at a higher rate [3, 5–7]. Stuttering is described as the observance of interruptions in speech fluency which may include repetitive sounds (one-syllable to words/phrases), prolongation of sounds, tense pauses, fixed postures of speech mechanisms, and difficulty in speaking [3, 6, 7]. Generally, as the child develops, the condition is usually self-resolved [5, 6]. However, if stuttering persists past the age of 4, risk factors to be explored are similar to those related to speech delay and include environmental factors such as home environment and traumatic events [3]. Great importance is placed on the early identification and intervention for stuttering in order to prevent long-term disabilities [6]. Referral to a speech therapist is highly recommended if the problem persists for treatment with syllable-timed speech and/or the Lidcombe Program, among other interventions [3, 5, 7].

# Behavioral Disorders

## *Aggression*

Aggression is often encountered in children as an expression of anger feelings, jealousy, and frustration. A certain amount of aggressive and/or assertive behaviors such as hitting, biting, and hair pulling is often considered a normal part of development [5, 8]. Frustration and irritability due to tiredness and mood variations among toddlers commence around the age of 15 months. It is at this age when toddlers experience expressive and physical limitations such as limited speech and slow mobility that awaken the feelings of frustration and irritation manifested as hitting, biting, throwing temper tantrums, and other aggressive behaviors [5].

## *Temper Tantrums*

Temper tantrums are sudden displays of anger, in which children experience an outburst of crying, yelling, and swinging of arms and legs and might be accompanied by hitting, biting, and pinching. Temper tantrums usually start around the ages of 15–18 months and persist until around the age of 4 years; however, they are most common at the age of 2, hence the popular nickname of the "terrible twos" [5, 9, 10]. The persistence of temper tantrums is affected by the parents' reaction.

To transform the "**terrible** twos" into "**terrific** twos" parents should be advised to try the following tips [5, 9, 10]:

- **Remain as calm** as possible. Shouting, yelling at, or hitting the child will not resolve the issue; it will only make the tantrum worse.
- **Ignore** the behavior when possible; this is especially effective when temper tantrums are a manifestation of attention seeking behavior.
- **Control and move** the child to a safe place; children who are hurting themselves or others during their tantrum need to be held firmly and talked to until they calm down. If the child is in a public place, she may be moved to a more private place such as the car or another room.

- **Distract** the child by shifting her focus on an item or an activity.
- **Look** at the child in the eyes and **talk to** her in a calm but stern manner in order to calm her down.

After the child has calmed down, the parents should also do the following [5, 9, 10]:

- Discuss the behavior with the child by talking about what happened and encouraging the child to express her feelings
- Explain to the child that throwing tantrums will not get her what she wants
- NEVER praise or reward the child for calming down from a tantrum

> ### *Advise*
> *When child takes something that is not his, try to gently say no and distract with another object –do not scold or punish*

> ### *Advise*
> *Children need to play with people and can learn from playing with brothers, sisters and friends*

## *Normal Versus Problematic Aggressive Behaviors*

Aggressive behaviors and tantrums become problematic when their frequency and intensity increase, as it is the case of a child who throws multiple temper tantrums per day, each lasting between 30 and 60 min or when those behaviors violate social rules and basic rights [8, 11]. High levels of aggression including harassment and hostile behaviors that are persistent over time present an increased risk for delinquency later in life [8].

Conditions that manifest as behavioral disorders include underlying intellectual disabilities, autism spectrum disorders, language delays, dysfunctional families, and ineffective parenting among others [8, 11].

Parents should be referred for professional counseling with a child psychologist and/or psychiatrist if the aggressive behavior is persistent and lasts for more than 6 months.

Table 4.1 below lists the manifestations of the most common behavioral disorders in children, namely oppositional defiant disorder (ODD) and conduct disorder (CD) [11, 12]. Early parental intervention is important in demonstrating appropriate social skills to the child and preventing antisocial behavior [8].

## *Picky Eating*

"Picky Eating," also known as selective or fussy eating, is used to refer to the habitual rejection of a large variety of foods among children [13–15]. Parents often recognize signs of picky eating when their children tend to consume a diet of limited variety of food only [13–15]. Picky eating may be observed from the age of a few months to well into several years [13]. This phenomenon is usually attributed to restricted and disciplined eating and seldom diagnosed as a clinical problem among children [13]. Distinguishing the underlying cause of picky eating is important for intervention purposes, because persistence throughout childhood may possibly lead to an increase in risk of overweight during adult years with consequent loss of self-esteem and wellness [13].

Children referred to as "picky-eaters" may suffer from underlying sensory processing problems, also known as **sensory integration disorders**, which result in feeding difficulties [14, 16]. Sensory integration disorders are neurological problems in which children are hypersensitive to sounds, light and dark, textures, and smells. In the case of picky eaters, they are most often sensitive to textures and tastes with certain aversions [13]. For instance, some children may refuse all foods with coarse textures such as grains and cereals, while others may refuse all foods with smooth textures [14, 15].

Signs of underlying sensory processing problems usually present as follows [13, 14, 17]:

- Gagging reflexes, vomiting, and/or coughing during meals
- Intake of a limited variety of foods

**Table 4.1 Most common behavioral disorders in children**

| | Oppositional defiant disorder (ODD) | | Conduct disorder (CD) |
|---|---|---|---|
| Four or more behaviors for at least 6 months | 1. Regular temper tantrums<br>2. Loss of temper<br>3. Arguing with adults<br>4. Deliberate defiance of requests<br>5. Deliberate nuisance<br>6. Angry and resentful feelings<br>7. Blaming others for misbehavior<br>8. Spiteful and vindictive actions | At least three behaviors demonstrated repetitively | 1. Aggressive behavior to people or animals: bullying; fighting; physical torture; use of weapons; forced sexual activity<br>2. Intentional destruction of property such as arson and vandalism<br>3. Deceitfulness: theft; lying<br>4. Violation of socially accepted rules in the child's environment |

- Difficulty during meal times (children tend to act out in order not to eat)
- Feeding time exceeds 45 min
- Hiding food in cheeks or under the tongue with refusal to chew

Parents are advised the following [13, 16, 17]:

- If the child presents with gagging and vomiting when trying a new food, do not insist on feeding and refrain from serving this type of food again
- If the child shows only aversion to a type of food, expose them to it once again at another time. Food may be paired with preferred food to increase acceptance
- Model eating certain types of food in front of the child without offering him/her any
- Refrain from entertaining or punishing children around meal times
- Refrain from refusing their children food at other times as punishment
- Seek sensory perception diagnosis and treatment for their children
- Discuss possible supplements with the doctor.

## Psychological Disorders

### *Attention Deficit Hyperactivity Disorder (ADHD)*

ADHD is a disorder causing problems with inattention, hyperactivity, and impulsivity [1, 5, 18]. Children with ADHD usually show impaired performance in school and aggression at home and among peers [1, 5, 18]. Symptoms can be observed as early as 3 or 4 years of age [19]. Factors associated with development of ADHD include attenuation of head growth percentile at 3 and 18 months, delay in motor development, behavioral characteristics, and delay in speech and language development at 9 and 18 months.

The diagnosis of ADHD is usually made around the age of 6 years when the symptoms become more apparent upon entry into an organized school system. ADHD symptoms appear as one of the following three subtypes [1, 5, 18]:

- *Inattentive* (previously known as Attention Deficit Disorder—ADD): The child has problems with focusing and attention, however is not overly active. This subtype is most common in girls and is usually unnoticed because the child does not usually cause disruptions.

- *Hyperactivity/Impulsivity*—The child exhibits hyperactivity and impulsivity in his/her actions, however does not have problems with attention.
- *Combined*—The child exhibits inattentiveness, hyperactivity, and impulsivity. This is the most common subtype in children with ADHD.

It is important to note that with time, hyperactivity among children with ADHD diminishes, however impulsivity and inattentiveness remain [1].

Conditions that may coexist with ADHD include [1]:

- Oppositional defiant disorder (ODD)
- Conduct disorder
- Anxiety disorder
- Depressive disorder
- Learning disabilities
- Sleep disturbances

Upon diagnosis of ADHD, treatments include medicines and behavioral treatment which focuses on parent and teacher training. Parent training helps parents learn how to interact with their children, understand their needs, and improve the abilities of their children for behavior self-management [1]. Parents need to be educated and followed-up on ADHD guidance for their children at home.

General tips that may be given during parental training include the following [20]:

- Give the child clear and brief rules to follow
- Assign the child chores in order to increase their sense of responsibility
- Use short checklists for the child to follow when assigning a task
- Maintain routines for meal times, homework, and stick to a regular schedule
- Offer incentives for behavior and praise the child for proper completion of tasks
- Minimize distractions around homework and chore times
- Stay close to child during tasks that require focusing (i.e., homework) and redirect his/her attention when distracted

**Table 4.2  Anxiety disorders affecting children**

| Type | Symptoms |
|---|---|
| Generalized anxiety disorder (GAD) | • Persistent generalized worry and excessive anxiety for a period of more than 6 months<br>• Fatigue and sleep difficulties<br>• Restlessness<br>• Difficulty and lack of concentration<br>• Irritability and muscle tension |
| Separation anxiety disorder (SAD) | • Excessive separation anxiety<br>• Impairs normal and healthy daily functioning<br>• Persistent for at least 4 weeks in children older than 6<br>*Separation anxiety is normal for infants under the age of 6, it only becomes a disorder if persistent and impairs healthy development and ability to function* |
| Social anxiety disorder (Social Phobia) | • Distress and fear of public and/or social situations for a period more than 6 months<br>• Avoidance of situations where embarrassment may occur<br>• Persistence of anxiety among peers |
| Panic disorder | **For a period of at least 1 month:**<br>• Unexpected panic attacks<br>• Distress and fear of occurrence and consequences of attacks<br>• Changes in behavior |
| Post-traumatic stress disorder (PTSD) | **Following exposure to a traumatic event, persistence of the symptoms below for more than 1 month:**<br>• Re-experience of traumatic events through dreams, recollections and re-enactment<br>• Physical and psychological distress in response to cues linked with the events<br>• Avoidance of thoughts, conversations, places, and people that may remind them of the traumatic event<br>• Avoidance of social interaction (isolation) |

## *Anxiety Disorders*

Anxiety disorders are characterized by pathological fear and anxiety that cause interference with healthy functioning and development of children [21, 22]. These disorders are the most common mental illnesses among children and are often associated with psychosocial impairments including inadequate social relationships, low self-esteem, and decreased academic performance [21, 22].

Special emphasis needs to be placed on diagnosis due to overlapping diagnostic criteria and symptoms with ADHD [22].

The different types of anxiety disorders affecting children include: generalized anxiety disorder (GAD), separation anxiety disorder (SAD), social anxiety disorder (social phobia), panic disorder and post-traumatic stress Disorder (PTSD) [21, 22] (Table 4.2).

Diagnosis of the above disorders should be made by a clinical psychologist or psychiatrist. Therapy may include cognitive behavioral therapy (CBT) and/or medications [21].

Therapy may often be supported at home through the adoption of the following techniques [5, 23]:

- Communication with the child to discuss fears and worries, identify feelings, help in problem solving by storytelling
- Creating and maintaining routines to establish a feeling of comfort and predictability and help in reducing anxiety
- Discouraging negative self-talk, challenging unhelpful thoughts, and encouraging optimistic thoughts and positive self-image
- Teaching relaxation skills to reduce stress
- Soothing and comforting the child

## References

1. Reiff MI, Stein MT. Attention-deficit/hyperactivity disorder. In: Voight RG, Macias MM, Myers SM, editors. Developmental and behavioral pediatrics. Elk Grove, IL: American Academy of Pediatrics; 2011. p. 327–48.
2. Smith PK, Cowie H and Blades M. Language. In: Smith et al., editors. Understanding children's development (3rd ed.). Malden, MA: Blackwell Publishers; 1998. p. 299–329.
3. Sharp HM, Hillenbrand K. Speech and language development and disorders in children. Pediatr Clin North Am. 2008;55:1159–73.

4. Macias MM, Twyman KA. Speech and language development and disorders. In: Voight RG, Macias MM, Myers SM, editors. Developmental and behavioral pediatrics. Elk Grove, IL: American Academy of Pediatrics; 2011. p. 201–19.

5. American Academy of Pediatrics. The wonder years (Altmann, tr. ed.). New York: Bantam Dell; 2007.

6. Conture EG, Curlee RF. Stuttering and related disorders of fluency. 3rd ed. New York: Thieme Medical Publishers; 2007.

7. Trajkovski N, Andrews C, Onslow M, Packman A, O'Brian S, Menzies R. Using syllable-timed speech to treat preschool children who stutter: A multiple baseline experiment. J Fluency Disord. 2009;34:1–10.

8. Smith PK, Cowie H and Blades M. Friends and school. In: Smith et al., editors. Understanding children's development (3rd ed.). Malden, MA: Blackwell Publishers; 1998. p. 109–140.

9. Harrington RG. Temper tantrums: guidelines for parents. National Association of School Psychologists Web site; 2004. http://www.nasponline.org/resources/behavior/tantrums_ho.aspx. Accessed 20 Jul 2011.

10. Temper tantrums – topic overview (2011). WebMD. http://children.webmd.com/tc/temper-tantrums-topic-overview. Accessed 18 Jul 2011.

11. Harstad EB, Barbaresi WJ. Disruptive behavior disorders. In: Voight RG, Macias MM, Myers SM, editors. Developmental and behavioral pediatrics. Elk Grove, IL: American Academy of Pediatrics; 2011. p. 349–58.

12. American Academy of Children Adolescent Psychiatry (AACAP). Facts for families No. 33: conduct disorder; 2004. http://www.aacap.org/galleries/FactsForFamilies/33_conduct_disorder.pdf. Accessed 12 Jul 2011.

13. Natenshon A. Understanding picky eating; 2006. http://www.empoweredparents.com/pickyeating/pickyeating8.htm. Accessed 26 Nov 2010.

14. Thompson SD, Bruns DA, Rains KW. Picky eating habits or sensory processing issues? exploring feeding difficulties in infants and toddlers. Young Exceptional Children. 2010;13(2):71–85.

15. Dovey TM, Staples PA, Gibson EL, Halford JCG. Food neophobia and 'picky/fussy' eating in children: a review. Appetite. 2008;50:181–93.

16. Natenshon A. Interventions for parents of children with eating and feeding dysfunction/picky eating, sensory integration disorder, and other brain processing disorders; 2010. http://www.empoweredparents.com/empoweredparents/pickyeating/consult.htm. Accessed 26 Nov 2010.

17. Chatoor I. Sensory food aversions in infants and toddlers. Zero to Three 2009;29(3):44–9.

18. Brain C, Mukherji P. Understanding child psychology. Cheltenham: Nelson Thornes; 2005.

19. Subcommittee on attention-deficit/hyperactivity disorder, steering committee on quality improvement and management ADHD: clinical practice guideline for the diagnosis, evaluation, and treatment of attention-deficit/hyperactivity disorder in children and adolescents. Pediatrics. 2011;128:1007.

20. American Academy of Pediatrics and National Initiative for Children's Healthcare Quality. ADHD – caring for children with ADHD: a resource toolkit for clinicians. Elk Grove, IL: American Academy of Pediatrics; 2002.
21. Spratt EG, Edwards JE. Anxiety and mood disorders. In: Voight RG, Macias MM, Myers SM, editors. Developmental and behavioral pediatrics. Elk Grove, IL: American Academy of Pediatrics; 2011. p. 359–98.
22. Anxiety disorders. WebMD; 2011. http://www.webmd.com/anxiety-panic/default.htm. Accessed 18 Jun 2011.
23. Eugster K. Anxiety in children: how parents can help. 2007; http://www.kathyeugster.com/articles/article004.htm. Accessed 18 Jun 2011.

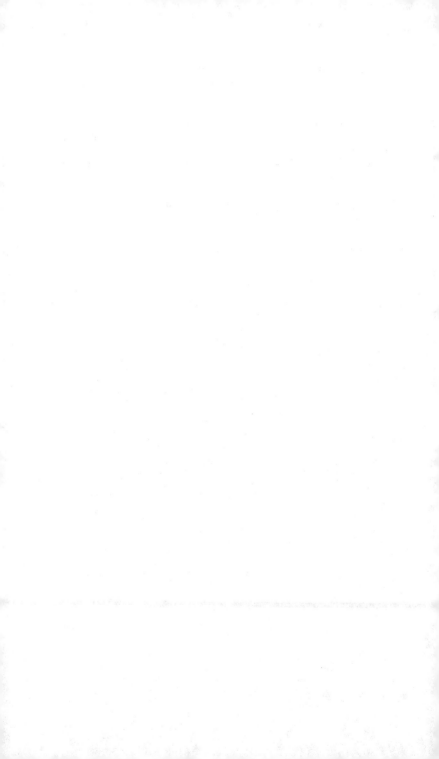

# Chapter 5
# Nutrition for Better Development

**Keywords** Health nutrition • Breast-feeding • Solid food • Vitamins • Bottle-feeding • Ketogenic diet • Glutin free diet

## Introduction

Adequate nutrition is crucial for the proper development of infants and children. Nutritional supplementation has shown clear benefits on the Development Quotient (DQ), which includes practical reasoning, eye and hand coordination, hearing and speech, and performance [1]. As seen in Fig. 5.1, stunted children who received a supplemented nutrition showed a significant increase in their DQ after 12 months compared to stunted children who were fed as usual for age [1]. This chapter outlines feeding guidelines in the developing infant and child as well as some special diets which may be indicated in certain conditions. In addition, developmental milestones pertaining to feeding will be addressed briefly.

## Breast-Feeding

Milk in general and breast milk in particular is the essential food for infants during their first year of life. Human milk is the most beneficial milk in the promotion of health, growth, and immunologic development of infants from birth and up to 2 years of age [2, 3]. Healthy

D. Sinno et al., *Enhancing Early Child Development:*
*A Handbook for Clinicians*, DOI 10.1007/978-1-4614-4827-3_5,
© Springer Science+Business Media, LLC 2013

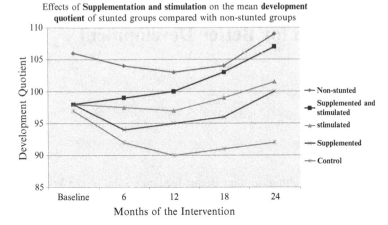

**Fig. 5.1** Effects of supplementation and stimulation on the mean development quotient of stunted groups compared with non-stunted groups. Reprinted with permission from: *The Lancet, 338(8758), S.M. Grantham-McGregor, C.A. Powell, S.P. Walker and J.H. Himes, Nutritional Supplementation, psychosocial stimulation, and mental development of stunted children: the Jamaican Study, 1–5, Copyright (1991)*

**Table 5.1** Sample menu—lactating mother (first 6 months) [6]

| Breakfast | Lunch | Dinner |
|---|---|---|
| • Orange juice | • Vegetable soup | • Green salad |
| • Whole-grain cereal | • Salty crackers | • Vinegar and oil dressing |
| • Banana | • Lean beef patty | • Broiled skinless chicken breast |
| • Whole-wheat toast | • Tomatoes, lettuce | • Brown rice |
| • Jelly or jam | • Fresh fruit salad | • Whole-grain roll |
| • Reduced fat milk | • Crackers | • Low-fat frozen yogurt |
| • Decaffeinated tea or coffee | • Reduced fat milk | • Reduced fat milk |
| | • Decaffeinated tea | • Decaffeinated tea |
| Midmorning snack | Mid-afternoon snack | Evening snack |
| • Fresh fruit | • Whole-grain crackers | • Reduced fat milk |
| • Bagel/toasted bread | • Cheese/Yogurt | • Medium apple |
| • Peanut butter[a] | • Fruit juice | |

[a]Avoid peanut butter if strong family history of peanut allergy

infants may receive their entire nutritional requirements exclusively from breast milk during the first 6 months of life [4, 5]. Moreover, preterm infants as well as sick newborns should be given breast milk as their primary source of feeding with very few exceptions [5].

The quality and quantity of breast milk production is influenced by the nutritional status and habits of the lactating mother [6]. The general recommended diet for a lactating mother involves an increased intake of calories, proteins, vitamins, and minerals. Lactating mothers should be advised to avoid dehydration and to drink around 8–12 cups of fluid per day according to their thirst feeling [6].

Table 5.1 represents a sample menu for a lactating mother.

## Developmental Milestones and Feeding

• Between 4 and 6 months of age infants' nutritional needs increase and supplementation with complementary feedings is needed to provide adequate amounts of calories minerals and vitamins. There are no clinical studies looking at the specific sequence or rate of solid food introduction at different ages. Infants differ in their readiness to accept complementary foods depending on their achievement of certain developmental milestones.

Following are developmental milestones that occur between 4 and 6 months of age and indicate readiness to solid food introduction [2]:

1. Fading of the extrusion reflex and ability to elevate the tongue to move pureed food forward and backward in mouth (extrusion reflex = tongue-thrust reflex that pushes food out of the mouth)
2. Ability to indicate desire for food, by opening mouth and leaning forward, or disinterest or satiety by leaning back and turning away
3. Ability to sit independently and to grasp foods with palms.

   • Between 7 and 9 months infants can start learning sipping from a small cup
   • Between 9 and 10 months:

- The pincer grasp or the ability to pick up finger food between thumb and forefinger develops
- Playing with a spoon at mealtimes without the ability to self-feed yet appears
- Holding of a cup or a bottle independently becomes possible

## *General Considerations*

1. Infants may lose up to 10 % of their birth weight in the first week of life and regain it by the end of the second week.
2. Feeding quantity varies from one infant to another and may vary in the same child between health and illness.
3. Microwave use for heating bottles or baby food should be discouraged because of possible excessive and heterogeneous heating resulting in burns.
4. Propping of the bottle against a towel to feed the infant should not be done because of the risk of choking.
5. When introducing solids, mothers should be advised to start with small feedings (e.g., two teaspoons), and to gradually increase until reaching actual needs.
6. Mothers should be warned from using bottles at bed time to avoid sleep association with bottle-feeding which might lead to dental cavities.
7. Mothers should be advised to introduce teeth brushing at an early age using a soft brush.
8. Mothers should be advised to continue full fat milk until 2 years of age, to switch to low fat between 2 and 4 years, and then to skimmed milk after 4 years of age [2].
9. Vitamin supplementation:

    (a) Breast-fed and preterm infants should be supplemented daily with 400 IU of vitamin D [2, 3, 5, 7]. Formula-fed infants should be supplemented if their milk intake is less than 1,000 ml per day.
    (b) Fluoride supplementation is recommended after 6 months if the fluoride water content is less than 0.3 mg/L (0.3 ppm) [3, 7].
    (c) Iron supplementation (1–2 mg/kg/day elemental iron) is recommended at 4 months of age for breast-fed infants. Formula-fed infants usually received adequate supplementation if taking iron fortified formula. Preterm infants should be supplemented with iron starting at around 6 weeks of age (3–4 mg/kg/day of elemental iron) [2, 3, 5, 7].

Table 5.2 is a suggested guideline for solid food introduction for different age groups.

## The Ten Yes's

1. Yes for exclusive breast-feeding up to 4–6 months of age.
2. Yes for gradual solid food introduction (one at a time) around 4–6 months of age.
3. Yes for feeding more during the day and avoiding night feeding after baby's weight reaches 5–6 kg.
4. Yes for paying attention to baby's cues of hunger and satiation.
5. Yes for regular meal times after 6 months of age.
6. Yes for putting baby in a high chair once able to sit without support.
7. Yes for involving baby during family meal times.
8. Yes for trying different food textures.
9. Yes for allowing baby to play with food and to feed himself or herself.
10. Yes for making feeding an enjoyable experience.

## The Ten No's [2, 8]

1. No white egg before 1 year of age.
2. No honey before 1 year of age.
3. No cow's milk before 1 year of age.
4. No spicy or hot foods before 1 year of age.
5. No Peanut butter before 2 years of age because of high risk of peanut allergy.
6. No finger foods that can cause choking (popcorn, grapes, raw carrots, nuts, hard candies, and hot dogs).
7. No nuts before 3 year of age because of risk of choking and foreign body aspiration.
8. No carbonated soda, no excessive fruit or sweetened drinks before 3 years of age.
9. No high calories food or "junk" food (chips, candies, chocolate, etc.).
10. No coffee or alcoholic beverages.

**Table 5.2** Feeding guidelines

| Age | Breast milk/formula | Cereals (AM snack) | Vegetables (Lunch) | Fruits/juices (PM snack) | Meat (Lunch) |
|---|---|---|---|---|---|
| 0–6 months | – Up to 10 feeds in breast-fed babies, less frequent in formula-fed babies<br>– 4–6 feeds at 6 months | None | None | None | None |
| 4–6 months | – Up to 10 feeds in breast-fed babies, less frequent in formula-fed babies<br>– 4–6 feeds at 6 months | Iron fortified rice cereal based on infant's development | Based on infant development | None | None |

| Age | Milk | Cereals | Vegetables | Fruits | Meats |
|---|---|---|---|---|---|
| 6–8 months | – Up to 4 feeds of milk per day | – Iron fortified single ingredient cereal (rice, maize, semolina, or wheat cereal)<br>– Later, follow by mixed cereals | – Start with one item at a time<br>– Blended baked or cooked vegetable (e.g., skinless potato zucchini, carrots, green beans, peas, avocado, broccoli, or spinach)<br>– Start small amounts and increase gradually<br>– Multiple ingredient vegetable soup at around 7 months[a] | – Start with one item at a time<br>– Blended, skinless (e.g., apple, pear, banana, carrots, melon, and peaches)<br>– Juices: unsweetened apple, grape, or carrot juice[a] | – After semisolid mixed vegetables<br>– Prepare vegetable soup in boiled meat water<br>– Meat may be added later, each kind at a time (chicken, turkey, or beef meat)[a] |
| 8–10 months | – Up to 4 feeds of milk per day<br>– Include cheese slices, and full fat yogourt/riocta cheese | – Mashed wheat and whole grain cereals<br>– Noodles, pasta<br>– Bread | – As above vegetables<br>– Add cauliflower and cabbage | – As above fruits<br>– Add mango, apricot, plums, and seedless grapes | – As above meats<br>– Add dry beans, fava bean[b], lentils, and chickpeas |

(continued)

**Table 5.2** (continued)

| Age | Breast milk/formula | Cereals (AM snack) | Vegetables (Lunch) | Fruits/juices (PM snack) | Meat (Lunch) |
|---|---|---|---|---|---|
| 10–12 months | Up to 4 feeds of milk per day<br>– As above | All types of cereals | All vegetables chopped and sliced into small pieces | All fruits. Use orange and citrus juices with caution in cases of allergy | Add egg yolk and fish |
| >12 months | 2–3 cups per day of milk or dairy products | All types of cereals, milk puddings | Semisolid family food introduced. Non-spicy | All types of juices | All types of meat |

[a]Introduce solid foods as a single-ingredient item at 2–7 days intervals to check for symptoms of allergy to any food item
Allergy may manifest as excessive crying, vomiting, diarrhea, or skin rash. [b]Do not include in diet if known G6PD deficiency

**Table 5.3** Average feeding quantities [2]

| Age | Daily requirements | |
|---|---|---|
| | Milk | Foods |
| 4–6 months | 4–6 feedings per day (150–200 ml of milk per feeding) | 1–4 teaspoonful of iron fortified rice cereal once or twice per day |
| | | After consultation of primary care pediatrician |
| 6–9 months | 3–5 feedings per day (no less than 850 ml per day) | 4–8 Table spoonful (Tbsp) iron fortified cereal |
| | | 6–9 Tbsp fruits |
| | | 4–6 Tbsp vegetables |
| | | 1–3 Tbsp meat or alternative |
| 9–12 months | 2–4 feedings per day (no less than 850 ml per day) | 4–6 Tbsp cereal (preferably iron-fortified) |
| | | 8–11 Tbsp fruit |
| | | 6–10 Tbsp vegetables |
| | | 4–6 Tbsp meat or alternative |

## *Suggested Feeding Practice*

1. Exclusive breast milk or formula feeding is recommended for the first 6 months of life.
2. To ensure an adequate amount of protein, fat, and carbohydrate during the next sixth to twelfth months, infants should be offered and should consume no more than an average of 850 ml of milk (28 oz) each day in addition to their quota of solids.
3. Different types of infant diets may be prepared according to age from Table 5.2 as examples:

Example

| | |
|---|---|
| Breakfast | Milk |
| Midmorning | Snack Cereals with or without milk OR fruits |
| Lunch | Meat, yellow or green vegetables plus 2 tea spoonful of oil, fruit OR milk |
| Mid-afternoon | Snack Cereals with or without milk C fruits |
| Dinner | Milk OR yogurt OR cereals with milk |
| Bedtime | Milk |
| Night | Milk (Table 5.3) |

# Specific Diets

## *Ketogenic Diet*

A ketogenic diet is a high-fat, low protein, and low carbohydrate diet mainly used as an alternative treatment for children with uncontrollable seizures [9–14]. The use of this diet has shown successful results for different seizure types, including refractory epilepsy [9, 10, 13]. Moreover, effectiveness has been demonstrated irrespective of frequency of seizures or age of the child [12, 13].

The ketogenic diet aims at maintaining a certain level of ketone bodies in the blood circulation (80–160 mg/dl) through increasing the intake of fat, limiting the proteins and carbohydrates one and forcing the body to burn fat [11, 15]. Studies have shown that a maintained state of ketosis induces an anti-epileptic effect, thus significantly reducing the frequency of seizures in children [9–13, 15].

A typical ketogenic diet is formulated according to a fat to proteins and carbohydrates ratio of 4:1 . This provides 90 % of the daily caloric/energy intake from fat and 10 % from protein and carbohydrate [10, 11, 15]. However, this ratio should be adapted to each individual case based on age and child needs [15].

## *Recommendations*

- This diet should be given under medical supervision [9, 15].
- A minimum of 3 months should be allowed to determine if the diet is successful or not [10].

## *Sample Ketogenic Diet*

*Infants* [13]
- Infants can have a formula made at home by mixing carbohydrate-free formula, with polycose–glucose polymers powder and micro-lipid fat supplement. This mixture has a similar taste similar to normal infant formula and therefore resistance to its intake is not a problem [13].

**Table 5.4** Examples of KD menu [15]

| Breakfast | Lunch | Dinner |
|---|---|---|
| • Scrambled eggs with butter | • Tuna with mayonnaise | • Broiled chicken breast |
| • Orange juice | • Celery and cucumber sticks | • Chopped lettuce with mayonnaise |
| • Vanilla cream shake | • Sugarless Jell-O with whipped cream | • Cinnamon apple slice with butter topped with vanilla ice cream |

**Table 5.5** Epilepsy syndromes and conditions where KD may be beneficial [10]

**Probable benefit based on at least two publications**
• Glucose transporter protein 1 (GLUT-1) deficiency
• Pyruvate dehydrogenase deficiency (PDHD)
• Myoclonic-astatic epilepsy (Doose syndrome)
• Tuberous sclerosis complex
• Rett syndrome
• Severe myoclonic epilepsy of infancy (Dravet syndrome)
• Infantile spasms
• Children receiving only formula (infants or enterally fed patients)
**Suggested benefit based on one case report or series**
• Selected mitochondrial disorders
• Glycogenosis type V
• Landau–Kleffner syndrome
• Lafora body disease
• Subacute sclerosing panencephalitis (SSPE)

*Older Children can have food supplemented with butter, mayonnaise, cream, sausages (Tables 5.4, 5.5, and 5.6).*

## Gluten-Free Diet

A gluten-free diet is a general diet in which all gluten-containing food is eliminated and is indicated for children with sensitivity to gluten [16, 17]. This diet is mainly used as a treatment for celiac disease [16–21] and in some instances for dermatitis herpetiformis

**Table 5.6** Contraindications to KD [10]

**Absolute**
- Carnitine deficiency (primary)
- Carnitine palmitoyltransferase (CPT) I or II deficiency
- Carnitine translocase deficiency
- β-oxidation defects
  - Medium-chain acyl dehydrogenase deficiency (MCAD)
  - Long-chain acyl dehydrogenase deficiency (LCAD)
  - Short-chain acyl dehydrogenase deficiency (SCAD)
  - Long-chain 3-hydroxyacyl-CoA deficiency
  - Medium-chain 3-hydroxyacyl-CoA deficiency
- Pyruvate carboxylase deficiency
- Porphyria

**Relative**
- Inability to maintain adequate nutrition
- Surgical focus identified by neuroimaging and video EEG monitoring
- Parent or caregiver noncompliance

Tables 5.5 and 5.6 reprinted with permission from: *Epilepsia, 50(2), E.H. Kossoff, B.A Zupec-Kania, P.E. Amark, K.R. Ballaban-Gil, A. G. Christina Bergqvist, R. Blackford, J.R. Buchhalter, R. H. Caraballo, J. H. Cross, M. G. Dahlin, E.J. Donner, J. Klepper, R. S. Jehle, H.D. Kim, Y.M.C. Liu, J. Nation, D.R. Nordli, Jr., H.H. Pfeifer, J.M. Rho, C.E. Stafstrom, E.A. Thiele, Z. Turner, E.C. Wirrell, J.W. Wheless, P. Veggiotti, E.P.G. Vining and The Charlie Foundation, and the Practice Committee of the Child Neurology Society, Optimal clinical management of children receiving the ketogenic diet: Recommendations of the International Ketogenic Diet Study Group, 304–317, Copyright (2009)*

[16]. Moreover, research is being conducted regarding its efficacy for children with autism and autism spectrum disorders [22].

Gluten is a protein found in wheat, rye, oats, barley, and their derivatives [16, 17, 20–22]. Therefore, a gluten-free diet is based on foods that do not contain any of the above listed ingredients. However, the exclusion of oats from this diet has been the subject of controversy [16, 17, 20]. Some studies have demonstrated the safety of including oats in the diet of patients with celiac disease [20], while others have argued that inclusion of oats may induce cross-reaction in the long term [16, 17].

Gluten-free diet has been found to decrease symptoms associated with gluten sensitivity such as diarrhea, distention, and flatulence [16], to promote bone growth, mineralization and maturation in those children with celiac disease [16, 18, 19, 21], and to improve biological functioning of children with autism [22].

**Table 5.7** Ingredients containing gluten [16]

| Exclude | Exclude until safety is established |
|---|---|
| • Wheat, rye, barley, kamut, spelt, and (for now) oats | • Modified food starch—may be derived from wheat |
| • Semolina, durum, triticale, graham flour, graham crackers | • Hydrolyzed or texturized plant or vegetable protein—may be derived from wheat |
| • Flour, self-rising flour, enriched flour, wheat starch, wheat gluten | • Brown rice syrup—may be made with a barley malt enzyme |
| • Cereal | • Seasonings and seasoning mixes—may contain wheat flour or hydrolyzed wheat protein |
| • Malt or cereal extracts, malt flavorings | |
| • Breading | |
| • Farina, bulgur | |

**Table 5.8** Sample gluten-free diet [16]

| Breakfast | Lunch |
|---|---|
| • Gluten-free toast | • 100 % pure-lean beef |
| • Orange juice | • Gluten-free bread |
| • Jelly or jam | • Gluten-free potato chips |
| • Reduced fat milk | • Carrot sticks |
| Snack | Dinner |
| • Peanut butter | • Chicken breast |
| • Fruit juice | • Boiled potatoes |
| • Gluten-free rice cakes | • Green beans |
| • Gluten-free ice cream | • Gluten-free bread |
| | • Reduced fat milk |

**Recommendations**

- Food product labels should always be examined carefully even when labeled as "wheat-free" are free of gluten [16, 17].
- Pharmacists and physicians should be consulted regarding medications that may contain gluten [16] (Tables 5.7 and 5.8).

# High-Calorie/High-Protein Diet

The High-Calorie/High-Protein Diet involves increased intake of protein and calorie dense foods with the aim of providing extra energy and nutrients to the infant in order to promote growth and weight gain and improve nutritional status [23]. The diet is recommended for conditions such as malnutrition, cystic fibrosis, failure to thrive, athetoid cerebral palsy, and many others [23].

For infants born with perinatal brain injury, high-calorie diet has been shown to increase brain and corticospinal tract growth, occipito-frontal circumference (OFC), and weight in both preterm and term infants [24]. Thus it is recommended for infants with perinatal brain injury, however results are restricted to physical growth and do not include improvements in cognitive function [24].

**Recommendations**

- For breast-feeding infants, supplements may be added to expressed breast milk in order to increase its caloric content [24]
- For older children (>1 year) the following foods may be used [23]:
  - Whole milk, cheese, and butter
  - Peanut butter, nuts, and seeds
  - Chicken, fish, red meat, pork, and eggs
  - Avocado, coconut, and dried fruit
  - Honey and sugar

## Omega-3 Fatty Acids

Omega-3 (n-3) fatty acids are unsaturated fatty acids which are essential dietary nutrients. Foods rich in Omega 3-fatty acids include seafood, walnuts, flaxseed oil, and fish oil supplements. Their benefits on various aspects of development include the following:

1. Improving cognitive and visual development after Omega-3 supplementation [25, 26].
2. Improving growth and function of nervous tissue after docosa-hexaenoic acid (DHA) supplementation [27].
3. Strengthening the immune system with prevention of allergy, infections, and other immune-mediated diseases after supplementation with n-3 long chain polyunsaturated fatty acids (LCPUFA) [28].

4. Improving memory function of school age children after supplementation with n-3 PUFAs of maternal diet or in early childhood [29].

### Recommendations [25–29]

- Inclusions of Omega-3 fatty acid supplementation in the diet during pregnancy.
- Inclusion of Omega-3 rich diet during solid food introduction in infancy.
- The benefits of formula supplementation with DHA remains controversial but may be beneficial.

# References

1. Grantham-McGregor SM, Powell CA, Walker SP, Himes JH. Nutritional supplementation, psychosocial stimulation, and mental development of stunted children: the Jamaican Study. Lancet. 1991;338(8758):1–5.
2. Promoting Healthy Nutrition. In: Hagan JF, Shaw JS and Duncan P, (editors). Bright future guidelines for health supervision of infants, children, and adolescents. 3rd ed. Elk Grove Village, IL: American Academy of Pediatrics; 2008. p. 121–145.
3. Slusser W, Powers NG. Breastfeeding update 1: immunology, nutrition & advocacy. Pediatr Rev. 1997;18:111–9.
4. Powers NG, Slusser W. Breastfeeding update 2: clinical lactation management. Pediatr Rev. 1997;18:147–61.
5. American Academy of Pediatrics Committee on Nutrition: Workgroup on Breastfeeding. Breastfeeding and the use of human milk. Pediatrics. 1997;100(6):1035–9.
6. Support for the lactating mother. In: Nevin-Folino NL, editor. Pediatric manual of clinical dietetics, 2nd ed. Chicago, IL: American Dietetic Association; 2003. p. 35–52.
7. Nutrition for the full-term infant. In: Nevin-Folino NL, editor. Pediatric manual of clinical dietetics, 2nd ed. Chicago, IL: American Dietetic Association; 2003. p. 55–72.
8. Hassink SG (2010). Getting started with solid foods. http://www.healthychildren.org/english/ages-stages/baby/feeding-nutrition/pages/getting-started-with-solid-foods.aspx. Accessed 21 Feb 2011.
9. Freeman JM, Vining EPG, Pillas DJ, Pyzik PL, Casey JC, Kelly MT. The efficacy of the ketogenic diet – 1998: a prospective evaluation of intervention in 150 children. Pediatrics. 1998;102(6):1358–63.
10. Kossoff EH, Zupec-Kania BA, Amark PE, Ballaban-Gil KR, Bergqvist AGC, Blackford R, Buchhalter JR, Caraballo RH, Cross JH, Dahlin MG, Donner

EJ, Klepper J, Jehle RS, Kim HD, Liu MC, Stafstrom CE, Thiele EA, Turner Z, Wirrell EC, Wheless JW, Veggiotti P, Vining EPG, The Charlie Foundation, and the Practice Committee of the Child Neurology Society. Optimal clinical management of children receiving the ketogenic diet: recommendations of the international ketogenic diet study group. Epilepsia. 2009;50(2):304–17.

11. Lefevre F, Aronson N. Ketogenic diet for the treatment of refractory epilepsy in children: a systematic review of efficacy. Pediatrics. 2000;105(4):e46.

12. Nordli DR, Kuroda MM, Carroll J, Koenigsberger DY, Hirsch LJ, Bruner HJ, Seidel WT, De Vivo DC. Experience with the ketogenic diet in infants. Pediatrics. 2001;108(1):129–33.

13. Rubenstein JE, Kossoff EH, Pyzik PL, Vining EPG, McGrogan JR, Freeman JM. Experience in the use of the ketogenic diet as early therapy. J Child Neurol. 2005;20(1):31–4.

14. Sirven J, Whedon B, Caplan D, Liporace J, Glosser D, O'Dwyer J, Sperling MR. The ketogenic diet for intractable epilepsy in adults: preliminary results. Epilepsia. 1999;40(12):1721–6.

15. Nutrition Management of Seizure Disorders. In: Nevin-Folino NL, editor. Pediatric manual of clinical dietetics. 2nd ed. Chicago, IL: American Dietetic Association; 2003. p. 423–49.

16. Gluten-Free Diet. In: Nevin-Folino NL, editor. Pediatric manual of clinical dietetics. 2nd ed. Chicago, IL: American Dietetic Association; 2003. p. 607–18.

17. Fasano A, Catassi C. Current approaches to diagnosis and treatment of celiac disease: an evolving spectrum. Gastroenterology. 2001;120(3):636–51.

18. Barera G, Mora S, Brambilla P, Ricotti A, Menni L, Beccio S, Bianchi C. Body composition in children with celiac disease and the effects of a gluten-free diet: a prospective case–control study. Am J Clin Nutr. 2001;72:71–5.

19. Kalayci AG, Kansu A, Girgin N, Kucuk O, Aras G. Bone mineral density and importance of a gluten-free diet in patients with celiac disease in childhood. Pediatrics. 2001;108(5):e89.

20. Picarelli A, Di Tola M, Sabbatella L, Gabrielli F, Di Cello T, Anania MC, Mastracchio A, Silano M, De Vincenzi M. Immunologic evidence of no harmful effect of oats in celiac disease. Am J Clin Nutr. 2001;74:137–40.

21. Tau C, Mautalen C, De Rosa S, Roca A, Valenzuela X. Bone mineral density in children with celiac disease. Effect of a gluten-free diet. Eur J Clin Nutr. 2006;60:358–63.

22. Whiteley P, Rodgers J, Savery D, Shattock P. A gluten-free diet as an intervention for autism and associated spectrum disorders: preliminary findings. Autism. 1999;3(1):45–65.

23. High-calorie/high-protein diet. In: Nevin-Folino NL, editor. Pediatric manual of clinical dietetics. 2nd ed. Chicago, IL: American Dietetic Association; 2003. p. 641–49.

24. Dabydeen L, Thomas JE, Aston TJ, Hartley H, Sinha SK, Eyre JA. High-energy and –protein diet increases brain and corticospinal tract growth in term and preterm infants after perinatal brain injury. Pediatrics. 2008;121(1):148–56.

25. Ayer JG, Harmer JA, Xuan W, Toelle B, Webb K, Almqvist C, Marks GB, Celermajer DS. Dietary supplementation with $n$-3 polyunsaturated fatty acids

in early childhood: effects on blood pressure and arterial structure and function at age 8 y. Am J Clin Nutr. 2009;90:438–46.

26. Innis SM. Omega-3 fatty acids and neural development to 2 years of age: do we know enough for dietary recommendations? J Pediatr Gastroenterol Nutr. 2009;48:S16–24.

27. Innis SM. Dietary (*n*-3) fatty acids and brain development. J Nutr. 2007;137:855–9.

28. Gottrand F. Long-chain polyunsaturated fatty acids influence the immune system of infants. J Nutr. 2008;138:1807S–12.

29. Boucher O, Burden MJ, Muckle G, Saint-Amour D, Ayotte P, Dewailly E, Nelson CA, Jacobson SW, Jacobson JL. Neurophysiologic and neurobehavioral evidence of beneficial effects of prenatal Omega-3 fatty acid intake on memory function at school age. Am J Clin Nutr. 2011;93(5):1025–37.

# Chapter 6
# Summary of the "Care for Childhood Development" Program (UNICEF/WHO)

**Keywords** Care giver • Early intervention • Stimulation • Learning • Communication • Family counseling • Check list

A group of experts in health, nutrition, and child development met at the International Child Development Centre (ICC) in Ankara in July 2007. They reviewed the WHO and UNICEF training for health workers, designed to improve counseling of families on child growth and psychosocial development in first-level health facilities in order to promote the healthy growth and development of young children.

The training could complement other child survival and health, nutrition, and early child care interventions in resource-poor areas, including programs to meet the needs of children living in communities affected by HIV/AIDS.

This chapter summarizes the manual developed by the World Health Organization (WHO) and UNICEF titled "Counsel the Family on Care for Child Development."

The chapter aims at:

1. Presenting to health providers skills which will enable them to identify interactions between children and their caregivers.
2. Counsel and advise the caregivers on activities to strengthen their relationship with their children and stimulate their growth and healthy development.

D. Sinno et al., *Enhancing Early Child Development:* 147
*A Handbook for Clinicians*, DOI 10.1007/978-1-4614-4827-3_6,
© Springer Science+Business Media, LLC 2013

# Who Is the Caregiver?

The caregiver is the person that is involved in taking care of the child's primary needs including feeding, communicating with and giving affection. Caregivers often have a strong relationship with the child due to their constant **interaction**. Mothers are the primary and most important caregivers in our communities to babies that are being breast-fed. Fathers and other family members may also be caregivers as well. It is important to build and maintain a good relationship with caregivers in order help them improve the lives of their children.

# Caring for the Child's Development

Care for child development is important because experiences during the first years of a child's life greatly affect their health as well as their communication and learning skills. Caring for children involves giving them love, attention, and opportunities to learn and develop. Families help their children grow healthier and stronger by playing and communicating with them.

Children begin learning at a very young age. They often learn through playing, observing, copying, and trying out what they see others around them do and often need a safe environment for that. While caring for a child, bear in mind that they **need consistent attention from at least one person**.

## *Learning at a Young Age*

Good nutrition and good health are important for the child before birth and during the first 2 years of life during the period in which the brain develops the most. Breast milk contributes to the development of the brain and strengthens the immune system of the child. Children can see and hear at birth and therefore it is important to stimulate their eyes and ears in order to develop their senses.

A clean and safe environment is also necessary for children to explore and learn new things and skills to avoid injuries and accidents.

Children often **explore** by putting objects in their mouths to learn textures and temperatures therefore attention needs to be given towards keeping only safe and clean objects around them. A safe environment is not restricted to protecting children from the physical environment but also from violence, anger, and criticism in order to provide them with confidence to explore and learn from around them. Caregivers may gently direct the child away from unsafe objects with a gentle "no" instead of harsh reprimand.

## Recommendations for Caring for the Child's Development

Communication and play activities are recommended to encourage and **stimulate** the development of physical, social, cognitive, and emotional skills of children (Table 6.1). The development of these skills is comprised of simple activities such as learning to reach or hold an object, stand and walk (physical); learning to communicate and express themselves (social); learning to think, compare, solve problems, and recognize objects (cognitive); and learning to be patient, happy, and to calm themselves when upset (emotional).

Promoting child development should focus on the care that the child receives rather than on the things that the child should be able to do at a certain age. The recommendations detail play and communication activities for children and their families. The activities provide the children with opportunities to learn new skills and help families learn to care for their children. These activities, couple with the basic care-giving skills of sensitivity and responsiveness, help caregivers respond to and provide better care for their children.

## Counsel the Family

The recommendations for play and communication can be used to counsel caregivers. Identifying problems in caregiving can be done through observing caregivers and their children. When meeting with a caregiver it is important to greet them and the child warmly and make them as comfortable as possible. Throughout the meeting, sit close,

Table 6.1 Recommendation for caring for child's development

| Newborn, birth up to 1 week your baby learns from birth | 1 week, up to 6 months | 6 months, up to 9 months | 9 months, up to 12 months | 12 months, up to 2 years | 2 years and older |
|---|---|---|---|---|---|
| *Play*: Provide ways for your baby to see, move hear, move arms and legs freely, and touch you. Gently soothe, stroke, and hold your child. Skin to skin is good. | *Play*: Provide ways for your child to see, hear, feel, move freely, and touch you. Slowly move colorful things for your child to see and reach for. Sample toys: shaker rattle, ring on a string. | *Play*: Give your child clean, safe household things to handle, bang, and drop. Sample toys: containers with lids, metal pot and spoon. | *Play*: Hide a child's favorite toy under a cloth or box. See if the child can find it. Play peekaboo. | *Play*: Give your child things to stack up and to put into containers and take out. Sample toys: Nesting and stacking objects, container and clothes, clips. | *Play*: Help your child count, name, and compare things. Make simple toys for your child. Sample toys: Objects of different colors and shapes to sort, stick or chalk board, puzzle.... |

**Communicate:** Look into your baby's eyes, and talk to your baby. When you are breast-feeding is a good time. Even a newborn baby sees your face and hears your voice.

**Communicate:** Smile and laugh with your child. Talk to your child. Get conversations going by copying your child's sounds or gestures.

**Communicate:** Respond to your child's sounds and interests. Call the child's name, and see your child respond.

**Communicate:** Tell your child the names of things and people. Show your child how to say things with hands, like "bye bye." Sample toy: doll with face.

**Communicate:** Ask your child simple questions. Respond to your child's attempts to talk. Show and talk about nature, pictures, and things.

**Communicate:** Encourage your child to talk and answer your child's questions. Teach your child stories, songs, and games. Talk about pictures or books. Sample toy: book with pictures.

**Table 6.2** Family counseling checklist scan

| All children | Look |
| --- | --- |
| | How does caregiver show he or she is aware of child's movements? |
| | How does caregiver comfort the child? |
| | How does caregiver correct the child? |
| **Child age less than 6 months** | **Ask and listen** |
| | How do you play with your baby? |
| | How do you talk to your baby? |
| | How do you get your baby to smile? |
| **Child age 6 months and older** | **Ask and listen** |
| | How do you play with your baby? |
| | How do you talk to your baby? |
| | How do you get your baby to smile? |
| | How do you think your child is learning? |

look directly at the caregiver and child, and communicate clearly. Information concerning the child and the caregiver and their relationship is gathered through asking the caregiver direct questions and observing his/her interaction with their child. The observations and the answers you receive will help in counseling the caregiver on how to encourage the child's development. The *Checklist for Counseling on Care for Child Development* can serve as a guide as you counsel the family (Table 6.2). The top of the checklist is mainly basic information that should be gathered about the child and caregiver. The middle part serves to gather information regarding the interaction between caregiver and child and the stimulation provided by the caregiver for the development of the child through communication and play activities. The questions in this part are divided into three sections: one section is to be used for all children, one for children less than 6 months old, and one for children 6 months and older.

*If a child appears to be weak and sick, caregiver should be advised to seek medical care and counseling should be deferred until the child is healthy.*

## *Family Counseling for All Children*

The questions in this section are based on the observations made during the counseling. The counselor should answer each question in a brief and concise manner, describing what he/she observed during the session.

- How does the caregiver show that he or she is aware of the child's movements?
- Many caregivers are unaware when they react to a child; however, small movements such as turning their hands with the child and looking the child's way when he/she moves indicate that the caregivers are aware of their child's movements. This **awareness of the child and reaction to his/her movements**, or connection between caregiver and child, is best developed when the child is very young. At times, caregivers may not be aware of the child and you do not feel a connection. There are many reasons including that the caregiver may be sick, tired, or separated from the child at birth.
- How does the caregiver comfort the child?
- Observe the response of the caregiver when the child is fussing or crying. Observe whether the child responds to the caregiver.
- How does the caregiver correct the child?
- Observe how the caregiver corrects the child when he/she makes mistakes or a mess. Actions may include scolding, punishing, distracting, or talking to the child.

## *Family Counseling for Children Less than 6 Months or 6 Months and Older*

The questions in this section are based on the questions asked during the counseling. The counselor should record the answers of the caregiver in a brief manner.

- Ask and listen: How do you play with your child?
- Some caregivers may think that their children are too young to play or that they only play with other children. Stress that the caregiver should **play with his/her child whatever their age is**.
- Ask and listen: How do you talk with your child?
- Some caregivers may think that their children are too young to talk to. Observe the caregiver's interaction with their child to point out

communication between them such as cooing or talking softly to calm the child is considered as **talking to the child at any age**.

- Ask and listen: How do you get your child to smile?
- Many caregivers find ways to make their child smile almost from birth. The child's responses to the actions of the caregiver encourage further communication between the two. Other caregivers attempt to force a smile out of the child by pulling their cheeks instead of gently encouraging a smile. Caregivers that do not try to get their child to smile have difficulty in responding easily to the child. Interacting with the child to have her/him **smile** is thus very desirable.
- Ask and listen: How do you think your child is learning?
- Most caregivers recognize when their child is having difficulty in learning, especially when compared to other children in the family or community.

## Improve Care Practices

### *Praise the Caregiver*

Praise to recognize the efforts of the family in doing the best for their children is important. It often encourages further attention on the family's part and helps in building the confidence of the caregivers to learn new activities for their children.

### *Advise the Caregiver*

Counseling families provides you with an opportunity to strengthen their skills in taking care of and understanding their children. Many caregivers may not know why their children do not respond to them and that they should talk to and play with them. The checklist identifies common problems and suggestions to resolve them.

- To help a caregiver respond to the child

With some caregivers, the close connection between their response and what the child wants is not apparent. There are exercises that can help teach the caregiver to look closely at the child and respond to him/her.

i.e., Ask the Caregiver to

(a) *Look into the child's face until their eyes meet*

(b) *Notice the child's every movement and sound*

(c) *Copy the child's movements and sounds*

Most children often start copying the caregiver's actions after the repetition of the exercise several times. The caregiver should be encouraged to repeat the exercises/games several times in order to strengthen their connection with the child.

**N.B: The counselor *should not* perform activities with the child directly. If the child connects with the counselor, it will interfere with making the connection with the caregiver. The counselor should limit his/her interference to teaching or coaching the caregiver throughout the activity.**

• To help a caregiver speak less harshly to a child

Some caregivers often scold and punish their children when they believe that they are misbehaving. Children often try new skills such as dropping and throwing objects, putting objects in their mouths, and so on. These actions **may be misunderstood for mischief**. It is important to point out to the caregiver the positive aspects of these actions by helping them see what their child might be thinking in a positive way.

**i.e.,** *"See what I can do. I can make it fall, and it makes a noise. The harder I push, the farther it goes. I am strong. When I drop it near Daddy, I am asking him to play with me, and we laugh and have fun together. He loves me very much."*

• To introduce a new play or communication activity

Introduce a new play or communication activity on the counseling card by following these steps:

(a) Get the child's attention—help the caregiver get the child's attention, for example, by looking into the child's eyes, smiling, and making sounds to illicit a response.

(b) Respond to the child—help the caregiver follow the child's lead by copying the child's sounds or responding to his/her hand or leg movements.

(c) Introduce a play or communication activity recommended on the counseling card—it is easier to introduce a new activity once the caregiver and child are **responding to each other**. Guide the caregiver through the activity—*keep in mind that as the counselor, you should not do the activity directly with the child.*

(d) State the recommendations on play or communication for the child— recommendations include tips on continuing and repeating the activity at home as well as introduction of recommendations for activities of older age groups if the child is at the end of an age group or already knows how to do the activities for his/her age group

(e) Check Understanding—make sure that the caregiver **performs the activity with the child in your presence**. Ask the caregiver questions on how he/she will do the activity at home and how often they plan on repeating it. Explain to the caregiver the importance of stimulating the child's development. The following reasons may be used:

- Play, communication, and good feeding in the first years of life will help your child become healthy and learn.
- Play and communication activities nourish the brain and help make your child smart and happy.
- Taking care of your child's development will help make them ready to go to school and become a productive member of the family and community when they grow up.
- Playing and communicating with your child helps you to build a strong relationship with them for life.

Some problems may arise when adapting the recommended play and communication activities at home. Ask the caregiver about potential problems they may face and help them identify appropriate solutions to these problems.

## *Child-Interaction Problem Solving*

**If the Mother does not breast-feed, counsel the mother to:** Hold the child close when feeding, look at the child, and talk or sing to the child.

**If the caregiver does not know what the child does to play or communicate:**

- Remind the caregiver that children play and communicate from birth
- Demonstrate how the child responds to his activities

**If the caregiver feels that she is too burdened or stressed to play and communicate with the child:**

- Listen to her feelings and help her identify a key person who can share her feelings and help her with her child
- Build her confidence by demonstrating her ability to carry out a simple activity
- Refer her to a local service, if needed and available

**If caregivers feel that they do not have time to play and communicate with the child:**

- Encourage them to combine play and communication activities with other care for the child
- Ask other family members to help care for the child or help with chores

**If caregiver has no toys for her child to play with, counsel her to:**

- Use any household objects that are clean and safe
- Make simple toys

**If the child is not responding or seems "slow":**

- Encourage the family to do extra play and communication activities with the child
- Check to see whether the child is able to see and to hear
- Refer the child with difficulties to special services
- Encourage the family to play and communicate with the child through touch and movement

**If the mother or father has to leave the child with someone else for a period of time:**

- Identify at least one person who can care for the child regularly, and give the child love and attention
- Get the child used to being with the new person gradually
- Encourage the mother and father to spend time with the child when possible

**If it seems that the child is being treated harshly:**

- Recommend better ways of dealing with the child.
- Encourage the family to look for opportunities to praise the child for good behavior

- Respect the child's feelings. Try to understand why the child is sad or angry
- Give the child choices about what to do, instead of saying "don't"

**Identifying children age 6 months and older who may be having difficulty learning:**

Ask the caregiver these questions:

*Hearing*

- Does your child turn his head to see someone behind him when the person speaks?
- Does your child show any reactions to strong or loud sounds?
- Does your child make a lot of different sounds (tata, dada, and baba)?

*Seeing*

- Does your child look at your eyes?
- Does your child follow a moving object with the head and eyes?
- Does your child recognize familiar people (like mother, father, brother, or sister)?
- Is your child able to grab an object?
- If the caregiver does not know an answer, ask to find out.
- For example, she can make a noise behind the child's head.
- She can see if the child's head and eyes will follow a moving pencil.
- For the caregiver to check the child's hearing and seeing, the child should be calm and not very sick.
- If any of the answer to these questions is "no," the child may have difficulties hearing or seeing. If special services for children are available in your area, refer the child for further assessment.

## *Follow Up the Caregiver and Child*

Following up with the caregivers is important. When caregivers have a follow-up visit, it often helps them start the new activities with their children faster. During the follow-up visit, ask the caregiver to show you what they have been doing with the child at home. Praise the caregivers for their efforts and advise them on additional activities.

# Index

D. Sinno et al., *Enhancing Early Child Development:*
*A Handbook for Clinicians*, DOI 10.1007/978-1-4614-4827-3,
© Springer Science+Business Media, LLC 2013